DEADLY SILENCE

DEADLY SILENCE

A Sister's Battle to Uncover
the Truth Behind the Murder
of Clodagh and Her Sons
by Alan Hawe

Jacqueline Connolly
WITH KATHRYN ROGERS

HACHETTE
BOOKS
IRELAND

Copyright © 2025 Jacqueline Connolly

First published in 2025 by Hachette Books Ireland

A CIP catalogue record for this title is available from the British Library.

ISBN 978 1 39970 665 0

Typeset in Sabon LT Std by Bookends Publishing Services, Dublin
Printed and bound in Great Britain by Clays Ltd, Elcograf S.p.A.

MIX
Paper | Supporting
responsible forestry
FSC
www.fsc.org
FSC® C104740

Hachette Books Ireland policy is to use papers that are natural,
renewable and recyclable products and made from wood grown
in sustainable forests. The logging and manufacturing processes
are expected to conform to the environmental regulations
of the country of origin.

Hachette Books Ireland
8 Castlecourt Centre
Castleknock
Dublin 15, Ireland

A division of Hachette UK Ltd
Carmelite House, 50 Victoria Embankment, London, EC4Y 0DZ

www.hachettebooksireland.ie

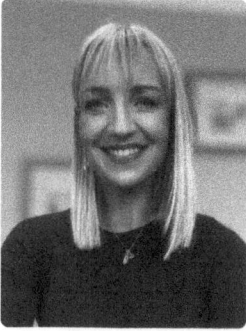

Jacqueline Connolly was born in rural Ireland and raised as one of three children. She works as a senior HR professional. She holds a master's degree in Human Resources Management and, inspired by her own experiences, has conducted valuable research into vicarious trauma, compassion fatigue, secondary traumatic stress and burnout for Irish healthcare workers.

She is an advocate for counselling, healing, and refusing to let catastrophe and adversity define us as people. As a result of her devastating loss, she is also passionate about raising awareness of domestic violence and the insidious nature of coercive control and other forms of domestic abuse.

She lives with her son in Cavan.

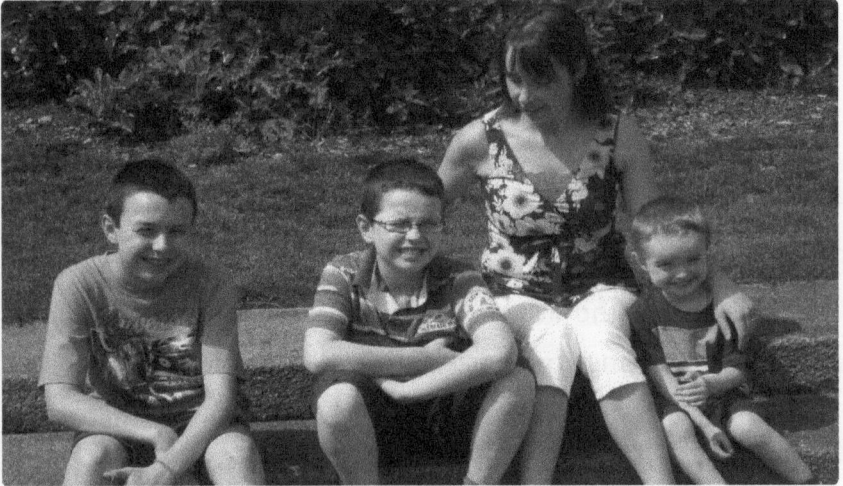

Clodagh, Liam, Niall and Ryan, this book is dedicated to your memory. Grief is love lost, and we've lost a world of love after your lives were so brutally stolen. We miss you all so much every day, but I know you are still with us, loving and protecting us.

I also dedicate this book to my mum, Mary, who is a constant source of love, resilience and strength. She is a wonder. Despite her pain, she has never lost her sense of humour and her ability to make us laugh and carry on.

This book is also in honour of every woman who struggles against domestic violence in all its forms. In memory of my sister and nephews, I hope to continue to advocate for more awareness, support and justice for all victims of such violence.

Contents

This book contains descriptions of domestic violence, murder and other distressing events. Some passages may be difficult to read. Reader discretion is advised.

Prologue

I have a recurring nightmare about the murders. I find myself walking through the back door of Clodagh's house. There is no lead-up to this. I don't know what has led me there. I enter the cosy family kitchen and feel overwhelming dread and panic when I see Alan Hawe before me. It feels so real.

His back is to me, and he's moving towards the door where my sister is. He hasn't seen or heard me, but I see him gripping the knife and the axe, and I know what he's about to do. I snatch something – sometimes it's a heavy pan. It feels solid and weighty in my hands, and I swing for his head. I strike him hard, and Hawe falls, the murder weapons tumbling to the floor with him.

I'm breathing heavily with the effort of felling him. He doesn't move again. I stare down at his crumpled form and relief rushes through me. I've saved them all – Clodagh, Liam, Niall and Ryan. In these panic-filled nightmares, I save them over and over again. I've done it countless times since they died. It must be my mind's way of coping, attempting to rewrite history. It's also probably a way of assuaging my guilt for not realising what Alan Hawe was capable of, for never spotting any red flags.

The nightmare always ends in the same way. I see Alan Hawe lying lifeless on the floor, and I know Clodagh is on her tablet in the living room, and the boys are upstairs, safe in their beds. That's when I wake up, and the real nightmare begins. I remember no one saved them, and I know I'll never see them again.

At times, finding justice for my sister and three nephews has felt as futile as my dreams of saving them. Mam and I set out with high hopes of learning the truth about why they died, but we're constantly fighting for progress. Our final meeting with the murder investigation team happened on 17 January 2019, and I still remember it as clear as yesterday.

We were brought to a room upstairs in Cavan garda station nearly two and a half years after Clodagh and her three boys were murdered by Alan Hawe. We had so many questions, and the list was growing. Just weeks earlier, on St Stephen's night, another issue arose.

My friend and I were in Matthews pub on Main Street in Virginia when a stranger approached me. 'Are you Jacqueline Connolly?' he asked.

I hesitated. I didn't know him.

'I want to talk to you about the night your sister and nephews were murdered.'

My heart sank. This was the last thing I wanted on a night over Christmas.

My friend Sinead leant in. 'Leave her alone. We're trying to enjoy our night out.'

We left the pub, but the man was persistent. He reappeared after we moved to the Riverfront Hotel in the town, insisting he had information I needed to know. I felt apprehensive, but I agreed to talk to him, standing under the camera outside.

He told me he had seen the murderer, Alan Hawe, the day the bodies were discovered. He said Hawe was driving his car.

'What time did you see him?'

'About half past six in the morning.'

By then Alan Hawe was supposed to have been dead for hours.

'Were you on your own?'

'No, I was with my cousin.'

'Where exactly did you see him?'

'Burrow Cross.'

I knew the Burrow Hill, but he told me where Burrow Cross was.

I asked other questions, including which direction Hawe was travelling. He seemed to have been on his way to the school where he was vice-principal.

'Did you report any of this?'

'I reported it at the time to a guard in Ballyjamesduff.' He gave me the garda's full name.

The man was adamant about seeing Hawe that morning, going to the guard and reporting it. He gave me so much detail that it seemed unlikely he was making it up. The gardaí had never mentioned the sighting to us. *What was Hawe doing on his way to the school that morning? Could he have been destroying evidence?*

For me, it was just another twist in a nightmarish story. Unfortunately, it could also have been another issue ignored in the investigation. I never realised that night that the truth would remain hidden for a further five years.

All I knew was the sighting of Hawe was inconsistent with everything we'd been told, but the case seemed full of inconsistencies. Hawe had told Clodagh he was concerned after seeing an envelope addressed to him on file in the school. It had not been found in the investigation. Could he have been going to the school that morning to destroy it?

Before I did anything with the information about the sighting, I messaged the same man the following day. He replied within minutes: I didn't tell you anything about seeing Alan Hawe that morning. I sat at the table, stunned, reading and rereading the message.

I pressed the heels of my palms into my eyes in confusion and despair. The first person I rang was Mam. I hardly knew what was going on any more or who to believe. This man's claims and his subsequent message had my head reeling. What was going on?

That was when Mam and I requested a meeting with the lead investigation detective via our garda family liaison officer. The meeting was granted in the New Year. For us, this 2 p.m. meeting with the guards was like a final opportunity to learn why Clodagh and her boys had died. We were tired and frustrated after two and a half years of asking questions.

Yet we felt anything but confident or determined as we travelled together from our homes in Virginia to Cavan town that afternoon. I felt queasy, and Mam was so quiet that I knew she was as nervous as I was. At the station, a guard told us to remain in our car until they had a room ready for us. We sat for a minute or two until one of us said, 'I'm not waiting in the car!' We were tired of being told what to do. We marched into the station but had to wait about fifteen minutes in the station's public office before being brought upstairs.

The garda investigation and the inquest had left us with more questions than answers. We still didn't know what had triggered Alan Hawe's murderous spree on the morning of 29 August 2016.

The letter Hawe left – we call it his 'murder letter' – and the evidence furnished by the investigation did not add up. Hawe said he was caught 'red-handed' and wrote that it would all 'blow up'. Who caught him red-handed, and what had he been doing?

I can still see Mam and me that afternoon in Cavan garda station. We sit opposite the lead detective of the murder investigation and a female guard in a room on the first floor. Behind the guards' heads, the windows look out over bare tree branches and across to Cavan courthouse on the opposite side of Farnham Street.

A long, broad conference table and growing mistrust separate us from the facing gardaí. The atmosphere in the room is as chilly as the winter day outside. Social niceties have been abandoned. No tea is offered.

Our family liaison officer is also attending the meeting. He sits to my right but remains silent throughout. Mam's voice is quiet and calm as she moves through our list of concerns.

'We've been going through his [Hawe's] letter,' Mam says. 'There are a lot of questions that were never answered, particularly around the area when Alan Hawe was caught masturbating in the school.'

I'm holding a document in my handbag that says this. It's a copy of the notes Alan Hawe's counsellor made. We need to know if this provides the answer – a trigger for everything that happened?

The lead detective and the guard glance at each other, and the former's response seems prickly.

'And where did you get that from?' he says.

'It's in the counsellor's notes,' says Mam. 'You have all of those, haven't you?'

'I don't recall anything in the counsellor's notes about [anyone] caught masturbating in school.'

'I have [his notes] with me,' I say. 'Do you want to see them?'

I indicate with a forefinger the line in the notes that reads, 'Alan masturbated somewhere he shouldn't have, possibly school.'

Before the discussion can go further, the female garda interjects: 'That's a garda report. Where did you get it?'

'Where did you get this?' echoes the detective.

'It was sent to the solicitor,' I say.

'What else did you get from the solicitor?'

I feel like I'm being investigated now.

'I have some concerns …' he adds.

'So do we,' I say.

'… that there has been a data protection breach.'

'We did not seek [the report and statement]. They were sent to us,' I say.

'Irrespective of all that, I have serious concerns about a data protection breach.'

'Well, my only concern is about my whole family that has been murdered,' Mam says, her voice low but clear in the room.

The meeting progresses, but we're facing a brick wall. 'We have investigated this to the nth degree …'; 'We have asked everybody …'; 'The answers we have got are the answers …'; 'We have done everything we can …'; 'If somebody saw Alan Hawe masturbating in the classroom, or whatever, we would have been told.'

The predominant concern of the gardaí in the room seemed to be data protection rather than the investigation.

'Have you any other statements in your possession at the moment?' the lead detective demands.

'Why are you making us feel like criminals?' Mam asks. 'There have to be lessons learnt from this. Otherwise, what is the point? It could be anybody's family tomorrow.'

We ask questions, lots of them. Mam and I have turned into detectives. *Was this looked into? Was that? Was Alan Hawe's car checked for blood?*

We discuss the people who have refused to give statements. The reply is, 'We can't force anybody to make a statement.'

I reach across the table and retrieve the garda report on the counsellor and his statement, which I showed the detective earlier.

'Jacqueline, I'm going to have to retain them, I'm afraid.'

'Why?'

'Because they are garda documents.'

'They were sent to us.'

'They shouldn't have been.'

'Well, that's not my fault.'

'Jacqueline, I cannot let you go out the door with those documents.'

'Are you going to arrest me?'

'No, I'm not.'

'Well, then, I'm afraid you're not having them,' I say,

shoving them into my bag. 'I brought them here in good faith to talk to you about them, and you're not going to seize them from me now.'

I suspect the detective's blood pressure is rising, but I don't care.

He raises the subject of the stranger who approached me in Virginia on St Stephen's night. He says this man denies ever talking to me. In the next breath, he wants to know if I had access to statements I shouldn't have. I can't understand why they're interrogating me instead of investigating the information that that man volunteered to me.

I can't help it. The frustration and stresses of the day are starting to take their toll, and I'm crying as I try to relate precisely what happened that night.

'He gave me all of those facts,' I say. 'He said he gave the statement to the garda [full name supplied] in Ballyjamesduff. Who would say something like that? I didn't make it up. He said he was with his cousin [full name supplied]. I didn't know him. I never met him before, so how would I know his cousin's name?'

But the detective still seems more concerned that I may have other statements in my possession. He says I am not entitled to have them. He talks at length about data protection regulation and the data protection commissioner. He seems worried that the guards will be fined.

We have gone way off track, far from Clodagh and the boys.

'With no disrespect, data protection is the least of our worries,' I say.

Mam says we may get answers if we go public with our story.

'Well, that's a matter for yourselves,' the detective replies. His tone makes clear that he couldn't care less. He just wants to ensure we have no garda reports that breach data protection rules. He wants to wrap up this meeting.

We persist. *Was this line of enquiry followed up?* We ask more questions. The lead investigator says he needs to check files or consult with other detectives to give us the answers we want. He'll get back to us. The meeting is at an end, and we have got nowhere.

'I would like you to leave with the assurance that every avenue was looked at, and we got every answer,' he says in conclusion.

So, more than two years since my sister's and nephews' murders, do we feel we've any answers at all? So much information needs to be uncovered and we suspect that more is being withheld from us.

I feel mentally and physically drained as we leave the garda station. I'm tired of the constant struggle, and my eyes sting with tears of frustration. But as we hit the cold air outside I find a new resolve. They will not defeat us. We will not go away quietly.

'This isn't over, Mam,' I say, as we head for the car.

Mam's face is set with grim determination. 'Not by a long way.'

This meeting with the gardaí is the turning point. We have been too quiet all along, hoping that justice would eventually run its course, and we would have the answers we need.

Instead, we were gagged at the inquest, onlookers in a public inquiry into the murders of our loved ones. We were warned that it would be adjourned if we asked a question.

The inquest revealed how my sister and my nephews were murdered, but no real questions were posed or answered. It seemed more of an exercise in protecting reputations while offering tributes to the victims and sympathy to the relatives. *Such an unimaginable tragedy, but let's move on now, folks.*

The garda investigation is over now too, and although everyone is coolly polite, we feel we're irritants to the guards. We still want answers, but they have done all they're prepared to do. We ask lots of questions. They say they'll get back to us. No one does. *Nothing to see here any more. Move on, ladies. The file is closed.*

It seems everyone is happy to spin a particular narrative of events: Alan Hawe was a devoted family man, a good dad, a loving husband, and a pillar of the community who snapped because of depression. He was a good man done down by temporary madness. The worst mass murder-suicide in Ireland was a family tragedy that couldn't have been avoided.

So much of the evidence points elsewhere. But the guards shrug because the perpetrator is dead. The thinking seems to be: *Sure, they're all gone. What's the point of looking into this now?*

Meanwhile Alan Hawe's words, written on the night he killed Clodagh and her boys, are etched in my mind's eye: *The truth would probably have come out some time.* That 'truth' remains concealed, and most seem content to let him take his dark secrets to the grave.

But we will not be silenced because we will never find peace of mind until our questions are answered.

Out of respect to Clodagh and Liam, Niall and Ryan, we must uncover the real facts about why they died. After all, if we don't fully understand why this happened, how can anyone stop it happening again?

I still dream about saving Clodagh and her boys, but I wake to the same nightmare: they are gone for ever. We owe it to her and her boys to uncover the truth and reveal the full story of their deaths. We also owe it to others living in the shadow of dangerous men, like Alan Hawe.

He may have extinguished their lives, but others who try to bury the memory of Clodagh and her boys will be met by our resounding defiance. They have been brutally silenced, but we won't be. We must be their voices now. This book is about breaking that silence.

1

Night Changes

What became hours of unimaginable horrors started as one of those glorious summer days when the sun casts a golden light over everything. That morning, of 29 August 2016, was even more hectic than usual. I had to get Gary, my son, dressed for his first day at preschool before getting to work. But as I dropped a bag of rubbish in the outside bin, a robin landed on the fence beside me. Robins are considered bad luck in some parts of the country. I distinctly recall eyeing the bird and thinking, *Please, go away*. I never see them as bad luck now. They're more like a sign from a loved one – little angels. They bring me peace.

As we left the house, I looked at Gary. 'You're so cute,' I said proudly. 'Let's get a picture of you.' I cherish that photo – Gary, with his big smile, standing at the front door in his new outfit of jeans, a long-sleeved T-shirt and sandals. I had no idea of the darkness that lay ahead.

I drove the short journey, hardly believing that Gary was already starting preschool. It was a milestone moment. My little boy was growing up.

The preschool was in a housing estate close to our home in Virginia, County Cavan. As we approached, he gripped my hand, but as soon as we went through the doors, Gary saw the throng of children and his face lit up. An only child, he loved any chance to socialise.

'I'm going to play, Mummy!' he said, dropping my hand and dashing straight in.

He was in heaven, scrambling over the multicoloured tyres in the garden and running around with the other children. I loved that Gary was so independent, but I was dabbing my eyes and blowing my nose as I embarked on the hour-and-a-half-long commute to work in Dublin.

As I drove along the N3, I thought about my sister, Clodagh, and kept an eye out for her black Renault Clio. After the summer holidays, she was returning to her job as a teacher at Scoil Chaitríona Naofa in Oristown, County Meath. She had a forty-minute drive from her Castlerahan home along some of the same stretch of road. I reached her turn-off for Kells without spotting her. I'd text her good luck when I got to my desk, I thought. I'd messaged her two days earlier. It was a meme with two monkeys on a tree branch. It read: *I smile because you are my sister; I laugh because there is nothing you can do about it.* I got no reply. I know now that Clodagh was being watched, and I was enemy number one in her husband's eyes.

I never did send her that good-luck text. My job as head of human resources in Clontarf Orthopaedic Hospital was busy, and duty called as soon as I got there. I was managing a co-worker in the office that day. Our only real chance for a break and a chat was to leave the hospital, so we strolled in the sunshine to Insomnia on Vernon Avenue for a coffee. We returned before noon, just as Veronica, a colleague from another office, appeared.

'I'd like you to come with me, Jacqueline,' she said.

I thought she wanted to discuss a meeting we'd had the week before. I explained I was busy and suggested we discuss whatever it was later.

My other colleague stood up to go. 'I'll leave and let you both talk.'

'No, I want Jacqueline to come with me now.'

Veronica was adamant, and I was irritated. 'Can we do this in the afternoon when I have more time?'

'No, Jacqueline. Come with me now.'

When I look back, I think, God love her. What must it have taken for her to maintain her composure as she attempted to bring me to somewhere private?

I went with her, not knowing where we were going. My office was in the old part of Clontarf Hospital. We walked past the canteen and along a corridor the length of the hospital. A couple of porters stopped me on the way. 'We need to talk with you, Jacqueline,' they said.

'I'll be with you shortly, lads,' I assured them. 'I'll come back to you as soon as I finish this.'

I didn't know what this was, and as the walk continued, I wondered, *Am I in trouble here?* When I asked Veronica what was going on, she didn't reply. Her heels clipped along the corridor. I remember glancing sideways at her several times as we made our way through the hospital, thinking her behaviour was bizarre. Finally, we got to the staff room used by the non-consultant doctors, and when Veronica opened the door, I saw the hospital's CEO, Michelle Fanning. Veronica didn't come in but pulled the door closed behind me.

I'm definitely in trouble, I thought. Michelle's office was next to mine upstairs. Why didn't she bring me into her office? What's going on?

Then I saw Leo Harrigan standing behind Michelle. Leo's mother, Edie, was Clodagh's next-door neighbour, and he owned a cleaning-products company in Trim. *Oh, he must be here for a meeting*, I thought. *Grand. I'm not in trouble so.* All these thoughts went through my head in milliseconds.

Leo didn't return my smile. 'Your mam is fine, and Gary is fine,' he said.

I felt a familiar tightness in my chest as my heart started pounding. No, no, not again. Please, God, not again.

'Who's dead, Leo?' I said, rigid with fear.

And then he started listing them.

'Alan, Clodagh, Liam, Niall and Ryan are dead, Jacqueline.'

What's he talking about?

I looked from Leo to Michelle almost accusingly, expecting one of them to admit this was some kind of sick joke.

'I'm sorry, Jacqueline,' someone said.

'You're lying!' I shrieked. The room spun. This made no sense at all. 'That's not possible. Sure, they don't even travel to work together. They don't go in the same car.'

'We don't know what happened.'

'No, this doesn't make any sense. I mean, this can't be true. You're talking rubbish!'

I recall this as a heated discussion, but colleagues told me much later that they heard my screams echo around the hospital. I remember Michelle saying they should get a doctor, but that was the last thing I wanted.

'I don't want a doctor. No doctor! I just want to go home. Now! I need to get home.'

Michelle rushed back to the office for my handbag and car keys, and I remember a fuss because they wouldn't let me drive my car. It seemed to take for ever to reach Leo's car and set off for Cavan.

I've no recollection of that drive from Clontarf Hospital to the toll booth at Dunboyne. I was lost in a fog of shock and confusion, and the journey down the motorway passed in a blur.

My first clear memory is getting to the toll at Dunboyne and ringing Mam.

'It's not true, is it, Mam? Sure, how could they be dead?'

I was in complete denial, and she was almost silent on the phone. She could scarcely utter a word to tell me what was happening. I learnt Mam was with her sister Carmel and her husband Gerry at their home in Oldcastle, Meath, but by the end of the call, I still didn't know what was happening with Clodagh.

I'll sort this out when I get home.

I always want to fix everything. I see that flaw in me. It took me a long time to realise that sometimes things are just too broken to fix.

There's some dreadful mistake, I thought.

I rang my friend Denise. 'It's crazy, Denise. They're saying they're all dead.' But she repeated the question I kept asking: 'But how? How could they all be dead?'

As Leo drove, I flicked through my phone distractedly. Suddenly a news headline jumped out at me, and I almost dropped it: Five Bodies Found in Co. Cavan Home.

I remember thinking, *This cannot be real. It just can't. This is some stupid misunderstanding*. Anyone not emotionally involved had no grounds to disbelieve what they were reading. However, shock was already exacting a toll, and I was in denial. They couldn't be dead, yet here it was, in black-and-white:

The discovery of the body of a man in his 40s, his wife in her 30s and their three sons aged 14, 11 and 6 was made at a house in Barconey, Ballyjamesduff, earlier today ...

I still didn't believe it. Even if something has happened, how could the media find out so soon? It's some kind of mistake.

Every emotion swirled inside me, and my stomach lurched. I wanted to get home. Someone would confirm this was all a colossal mistake. Clodagh might even have returned and explained how the vile rumour had started.

Carmel and her husband live about eleven kilometres from my mother's house and mine in Virginia, and I knew the route like the back of my hand. But that day, I didn't know where I was and became confused on the side roads. I was in some kind of fog and couldn't direct Leo to the house. We drove and drove. The journey seemed interminable, and I recall trembling with cold even though the sun beat down on the car.

The bright weather always stands out in stark contrast to the darkness of that day. Even today, years later, it's difficult to enjoy sunny days like I used to, especially when I hear the excited shrieks of children playing. Those sounds are a constant reminder that Clodagh's boys will never see sunshine again.

2

Clodagh, Liam, Niall and Ryan's Last Day

I couldn't process what was going on. My sister Clodagh, four years older than me, was a loving mother, and a rock of good sense. Her husband, Alan, was the epitome of responsibility. I never warmed to him. I thought he was boring, but for Clodagh's sake, I tried. Despite my efforts, I always struggled to make conversation with him so avoided him when I could. But as a parent, I thought he would die to protect their children. Both parents were fiercely protective and proud of their boys, Liam (fourteen), Niall (eleven) and Ryan (six).

That day, it seemed impossible they could be dead. My head was spinning, as I tried to figure out what had happened. They couldn't have died in a car accident. Alan was vice-principal of Castlerahan National School, which he could see across the fields from their house. A three-minute drive down a country lane brought him and the youngest two boys to the school gates. Clodagh was the only one with a more significant drive to Kells.

Were they sick? Did something poison them? Could there have been some kind of row? I dismissed the latter notion almost as soon as I thought of it. Alan and Clodagh were an incredibly close couple. It made no sense. My priority was to see Mam. I had to get home and clear this up.

Leo pulled up outside my aunt and uncle's house, and I remember walking through their door into an eerie silence. That was the first time I thought the impossible might be true. Nobody could speak. I have a memory of my cousin Melissa meeting my gaze with red-rimmed eyes from the sunroom. After that, I have brief flashbacks of that day: Mam and Carmel walking the garden in circles, and Mam saying, 'Alan has done something terrible.'

I've never forgotten her words because they came as a terrible jolt. That was when I realised this wasn't a mistake. Yet, still, their deaths didn't feel real to me.

I mostly remember the silence. There were no words to express what we were going through. And no one called. I expected gardaí to arrive at any minute to tell us what was happening, but they didn't come.

Mam was almost catatonic with shock. It was hours before

she could even form the words to tell us that Alan had left a note on the back door. To be honest, I'm not sure what I heard that day and what I absorbed over the following days and weeks. Slowly, we learnt the sequence of events leading up to Clodagh and her boys' deaths.

Liam had had a basketball match in Virginia the previous evening. She, Alan and the other two boys had attended the Sunday game. Alan, who was treasurer of Castlerahan GAA club, was out collecting for the club the same day. After the game, around half past six or seven o'clock, they called into Mam's house.

I wasn't there because it was my late husband Richie's birthday. I marked the occasion by going to the grave, then spending the day with our son, Gary. Clodagh hadn't sent a text, and by that evening, I was a little annoyed that she hadn't acknowledged the date. I feel guilty now for that.

Mam thought everything between Alan and Clodagh appeared normal. Alan looked up a few things for Mam on her computer – the Lotto numbers and dates for the National Ploughing Championships. We all knew Alan was having a few problems at his school, and Mam said something about one of his colleagues out of his earshot. Clodagh dropped her voice and said, 'Don't mention that name in front of Alan.'

Otherwise, it was another pleasant but ordinary family gathering, a grandmother with her daughter, son-in-law and grandchildren. The adults had tea and biscuits in the kitchen, and the boys sat in front of the telly with crisps.

Ryan was delighted to get his favourite salt and vinegar flavour. (Mam retrieved the empty packet afterwards and still holds on to it.) Alan was due to attend a staff meeting at his school the next day, but classes wouldn't start for pupils until Tuesday. As Niall and Ryan wouldn't have school, Clodagh arranged to drop them at Mam's on her way to work the following morning.

Mam and the boys made plans to pick blackberries, and Niall, a budding baker, looked forward to making blackberry and apple crumble with his granny. They left Mam's before 9 p.m. as Clodagh said she still had to bath Ryan before bed.

Mam knew Alan wasn't looking forward to returning to school, so she wished him luck as he left. 'Thanks for the goodies, Mary,' he replied. And that was it. There were no red flags, nothing untoward, just an ordinary evening with tea and biscuits and chat and the three boys eating crisps in front of the TV.

Much later, when we pressed her, all Mam could remember that was out of the ordinary was Alan using the bathroom in her house. It sounds daft, but he never used anyone else's bathroom. It was just a quirk of his we'd noticed down the years. But that was all she could think of. Apart from that unremarkable detail, it was just another family evening, like many others before it.

The following morning, Mam waited for Clodagh to drop off the two boys on her way to school. She expected them at around 8.30 a.m., but as time ticked on, she became concerned. Clodagh always called when she was going to be late. Mam tried calling Alan's mobile phone, the house phone and Clodagh's mobile. She sent a few texts. When no one answered or called her back, she knew something was wrong. She got into her car and drove to their place.

Clodagh lived in a red-brick dormer home in Oakdene Downs, a residential close of four modern detached houses in rural Cavan countryside. The house is in a lovely spot, on an elevated site off a winding country road. They were surrounded by views of the fields and trees, and were a three-minute drive from Castlerahan's church and national school.

Castlerahan is in the centre of a triangle between Oldcastle, Virginia and Ballyjamesduff. The drive from Mam's house in Virginia took less than ten minutes. When she pulled into the quiet estate, Mam grew even more concerned. She saw Alan and Clodagh's cars parked in the driveway, and the curtains were still drawn.

Mam's immediate worry was a carbon-monoxide leak, so she hurried around to the back door and was about to unlock it with her key. She spotted a note in Alan's handwriting. It warned: 'Don't come in. Call the gardaí.'

For my own sake alone, I thank God she never went in there. I know in my heart she wouldn't be here now if she had witnessed the scene inside. Mam lived with Clodagh and Alan when she first moved to Virginia. If the timing had been different and she had been there that night, she probably wouldn't be here now either. Clodagh had tried to persuade

Mam to live with them, promising to build onto their house for her, but Mam, an independent woman, had said no. There is no doubt in my mind Alan Hawe would have had a fifth victim. I feel grateful to have her here.

When she saw that note on the door, Mam was trembling so much it took several attempts to dial 999. She ran next door to the neighbour, Edie Harrigan and told her what she later told us – that she thought Alan had done something terrible.

Gardaí Alan Ratcliffe and Aisling Walsh from Bally-jamesduff station were the first to enter the house. Minutes later, Garda Ratcliffe emerged to break the news to Mam that no one was left alive. Mam's entire world fell apart.

That was it. We knew nothing else, only that they were all dead. Any conversation we had that day consisted of expressions of disbelief. We said over and over that Alan loved Clodagh and his boys: something terrible must have happened to him, and he must have snapped.

We waited all that afternoon, expecting to hear from gardaí. They had my mother's number, but no one called. I remember googling local priests and ringing Father Felim Kelly in Clodagh's parish, but there wasn't a priest to be found in Castlerahan. Instead, our priest from Virginia called the next day to offer spiritual support.

That evening Gerry took a call from the guards. They wanted to know if we wished to go to Clodagh's house before they brought the bodies to the mortuary at Our

Lady of Lourdes hospital in Drogheda. My work brings me there from time to time, and I think about Clodagh and her boys every time I park outside. Mam hesitated about going to the mortuary. She didn't know if she wanted to see their bodies.

'I'm going,' I said, standing up. I thought maybe their loss might feel real if I went to the house.

Gerry looked worried. 'The gardaí say there's a lot of media surrounding the house,' he said. 'They're waiting by the gate, and they're in the fields. They said photographers are standing on the walls around the estate.'

We were a private family and had never had any media experience. Attention like this was terrifying. We felt raw and emotional enough without that kind of exposure. I feared there would be a media frenzy if we went to the house, and we could hardly bear to talk about what had happened with each other, never mind with strangers. I decided not to go.

My car was still in Dublin, so my cousin Melissa collected Gary from preschool, and that evening, Mam, Gary and I went to my house in Virginia. It seemed like an entirely different house from the bright and cheerful home I'd left that morning.

That night I was exhausted but couldn't sleep. Next morning, I rose to face the same heavy air of disbelief, shock and eerie quiet. I felt nauseous but had to muster the energy to appear cheery and normal for my little boy's sake.

Later that morning, Mam told me for the first time about Alan Hawe's obsession with pornography. When Clodagh had confronted him about it, he claimed he had been looking at images of women naked 'from the waist up', as he put it. Clodagh had told Mam he was seeing a counsellor to discuss it.

It didn't sound serious, but it shocked me because this was Alan: bland, boring but reliable Alan. And because I thought Clodagh had a rock-solid marriage. I never suspected they had any problems.

Some couples include pornography in their relationship, but when it is used in secrecy, it can be devastating to a partner. I understood that this would be an issue for Clodagh. She was half of an all-consuming marriage. She and Alan never went to the pub or socialised with other people, apart from immediate family. She didn't do anything outside her family or have separate interests from Alan or her children. Clodagh and Alan's lifestyle was insular. Discovering her husband was watching pornography must have felt like a huge betrayal. He was filling a void by exploiting strangers rather than embracing the real love around him.

She believed she was part of a very intense, very close partnership. His attraction to pornography must have made her feel she was not good enough. It must have crushed her belief in their bond as a couple, but she did her best to overcome their problems, especially as he had agreed to get professional counselling. Of course, the pornography

Alan admitted to watching was so far removed from the reality that Clodagh had no idea what was going on. But we wouldn't learn that for a long time.

I was sorry to hear that Clodagh had been having marriage problems. But once I got over the initial shock of discovering Alan was in therapy for looking at pornography, I thought it wasn't hugely significant. Of course, I understood Clodagh's sense of hurt. But at least Alan had been trying to resolve their problems by seeing a counsellor.

I still couldn't conceive of why or how he killed them all. I was convinced that the only explanation for what happened was that he had some sort of terrible mental breakdown.

That day, the gardaí assigned a family liaison officer to us, but we heard nothing more about what had happened in that house. We heard very little from anyone else either. Usually, with a death in the family, the doorbell rings all the time with offers of food and sympathy. It seemed no one else could cope with the news either. They might not have known how to react or were afraid of saying the wrong thing, but it was as if the magnitude of what had happened had made us pariahs. We felt isolated in our suffering.

We had been trying to contact the Hawe family since the day before. We had hoped that Alan's dad, Stephen, or his brother, PJ, might officially identify the bodies, so we rang and left a message but didn't hear back. Instead, Gerry had to identify Clodagh, Liam, Niall, Ryan and Alan Hawe.

To this day, I can't imagine what that was like for him or

how he dealt with it. He loved Clodagh and those children. A true hero, he has never spoken about it. I should have done it, but couldn't face looking upon the lifeless bodies of my sister and my three little nephews in a mortuary.

That evening, more than a day and a half after their bodies were discovered, we still knew nothing about what had happened to them. I resorted to reading articles online to glean whatever information I could. That was when I stumbled upon a report that made me gasp and recoil from the screen. A newspaper headline said Clodagh had been murdered with a hatchet.

I read it aloud, and we looked at each other in horror, then went into complete denial. No! The media are making this up … sensationalising things …That never happened. They can't write stuff like that, surely?

I'd thought things couldn't get any worse after I'd been told Clodagh, Alan and the boys were dead. I had no idea what was coming.

3

Home

Clodagh and I grew up watching our parents' marriage unravel around us. We seemed to gravitate towards each other as they drifted to opposite ends of the house. Clodagh was four years older, but she and I couldn't have been closer during those years. Our bond strengthened even further as our relationship with our father fractured.

In February 1994, Mam insisted on making a big fuss over my thirteenth birthday. She always made our birthdays wonderful so we felt special and loved.

Mam was honest with us, so she told us when Granddad, her father, became seriously ill. Things were fraught between herself and Dad too, so my birthday was the perfect opportunity to lift all our spirits. She bought me a musical box in a colourful strawberry print that I still treasure. I keep inside it a pillbox that Granddad gave me, containing two Panadol (never resorted to when hung-over).

I remember Mam lined up my birthday cards – some adorned with tin badges reading: 'Now You Are 13' – on the kitchen windowsill. Then she laid a feast of treats on the table, including an iced birthday cake adorned with thirteen multi-coloured candles. Clodagh and our little brother, Tadhg, three years younger than me, sang a rousing chorus of 'Happy Birthday'. I beamed, loving all the attention, and blew out my candles to applause. Dad wasn't there, of course.

He was in the kitchen a couple of days later. The window was open, and a sudden draught whipped the birthday cards into the garden. 'Someone's cards flew out the window,' he remarked, as he buttered bread.

Someone's cards. That comment hurt: he hadn't even wished me a happy birthday. I remember getting up from the table and running to my room, choking with tears. Mam overheard what he said, so she ran after me, but I was inconsolable.

A week later, Granddad died, and I felt even more bereft. His home up the road was a warm hug and a safe harbour in the storm of my parents' marriage breakdown. I spent many evenings sitting with him at his front door while he scared me witless relating stories about banshees. I remember enquiring about the bottle of water always kept in his bedroom.

'It's holy water. Take a drink and clear all your sins,' he said. I tipped back the bottle and gasped at the rush of heat that hit the back of my throat. Poitín. My first sip of alcohol was illegal hooch. I'll always remember Granddad rocking with laughter as Mam gave him a bollocking afterwards. I adored him and felt adrift without his presence.

The breakdown of my parents' marriage and the constant tension in the house cast a long shadow over my childhood. Most painful for me was the disintegration of my relationship with my father. Clodagh shadowed Mam, but I was a daddy's girl growing up. I adored him, trailing around after him whenever I could.

Our family home, in rural Clontyduffy, near Mountnugent in Cavan, was surrounded by rolling hills, fields, hedgerows and cattle. We lived in a large four-bedroom modern dormer bungalow with my dad's carpentry workshop built behind it.

I was thrilled whenever he let me join him in the van as he went on carpentry jobs around the county. Sometimes, he'd stop and buy me a Cadbury Creme Egg as a treat, and I'd lick the insides hollow, the melting chocolate smearing my hands and face. I cherished the treat even more because it was just for me – not for Mam, Clodagh or Tadhg.

In the mid-nineties in Ireland, considerable stigma was associated with marriage breakdown. I didn't know of anyone else in school with parents who were separated. Like any teenager, I longed to be the same as everyone else, so my home life was largely a secret.

As I got older and could understand more of what was going on, I grew more disenchanted with my father. My parents were separated but still living in the same house. I watched as he drifted in and out of our lives, sometimes disappearing for days. Mam worked long hours as a nurse to keep us and get us all through school. Mam, Clodagh, Tadhg and I became a team, living apart from our father but still under one roof. Dad did his thing, and we did ours.

As my father distanced himself, I felt rejected. I was young, vulnerable and began harbouring resentment towards him. Dad catered for himself, buying his own groceries. I started eating his food, especially his store of cakes and biscuits, to make him angry and get his attention. However, if he noticed, he never said.

After a few months of doing that, I discovered I was piling on weight. That didn't stop me eating his food – I started vomiting it. I was in emotional turmoil and angry with my father so I took it out on myself. My way of coping with the chaos and distress I felt was to control one of the few things I could – what I ate. That was the start of my unhealthy relationship with food. From then on, cycles of starving or purging would begin whenever I felt stressed.

Not much happened in Clontyduffy so, as kids, Clodagh and I had to amuse ourselves as best we could. As sisters, we were very close, and we adored Tadhg. We used to love dressing him up in outfits to make him look like a little prince. He wouldn't thank me for saying this, but we treated him as our living doll.

I remember Clodagh going around in a plaster cast up one leg because of a knee injury. We were wandering the fields, and I don't know what came over her, but Clodagh tried to cross an open drain in a field of cattle. Unfortunately, her plaster of Paris leg sank in the drain right up to her knee, and she couldn't yank herself out. Poor Clodagh was stuck in two feet of cow shit, and I laughed so hard that I couldn't help her out. An incident like that was the height of entertainment for kids in Clontyduffy in those days.

Growing up, I was never conscious of the four-year age gap between Clodagh and me. But when things were going badly with Mam and Dad, Clodagh was a protective presence, taking Tadhg and me away from the crossfire and distracting us. Clodagh was always the 'good' girl at home. She was studious and responsible. She looked out for all of us.

When Clodagh was seventeen, she left home to start teacher training at St Patrick's College in Drumcondra, Dublin. The day she left, she and Dad had an exchange of words. After that she had little communication with him, refusing to come home while he was there, and never made up with him. He never met Alan Hawe or his three grandchildren.

Life at home the year after Clodagh left was horrendous, and I felt lost without her. I wasn't speaking to my father. I started going to Dublin to stay with Clodagh the odd weekend. We'd go to the cinema or shopping, and I remember dreading Sundays when I'd have to leave her and go home.

Dad finally left home the year after Clodagh went to college, on Christmas Eve 1995. It should be devastating to have a parent leave on Christmas Eve. For me, it felt like a huge weight had been lifted, and I could breathe for the first time in years. The atmosphere at home was transformed overnight, and Clodagh started staying again.

Mam never made us choose between her and Dad and always said we could see our father anytime. Tadhg was only about eleven when Dad left, and they stayed in touch for a long time, but I had no communication with him for many years.

4

The Best Brother

Clodagh dated a guy in college for a brief spell. The only memorable thing about him was that he chose to break up with her on Valentine's Day. Shortly afterwards, she met Alan Hawe, and that was it. She was still in her first year in teacher training, and they lived on campus but in separate houses. He knew all the right words. Early in their relationship, he told her, 'I'll always look after you, Clodagh.'

Clodagh couldn't have been happier as she related his words to us. They were the magic words my sister must have longed to hear after all she had been through. She had eyes for no one else.

Alan didn't drink or go to the pub. He was reliable, faithful, sensible and studious. He believed in God, marriage, family and traditional values. Alan was everything our father wasn't, and I truly believe that childhood trauma influences so many decisions later in life.

For Clodagh, none of the usual rites of passage marked her transition into adulthood: no sowing of wild oats or party-crazy student days. Instead, Alan was Clodagh's first serious boyfriend, and while she enjoyed an occasional drink before she'd met him, she never drank afterwards.

Our first and most significant falling out as sisters happened after she'd met Alan Hawe. They were still students in St Patrick's, and he was travelling from his family home in Windgap, County Kilkenny, to our house for the weekend.

It wasn't his first visit to us, but it was a blustery winter's night and Clodagh was worried about him driving. She was up and down, standing by the window, twitching the curtains and watching anxiously for him. The house phone rang every so often as Alan called from a phone box to relay his latest progress and reassure Clodagh that he was still safe. I rolled my eyes as this went on. It seemed like a lot of drama over a two-hour drive. But Clodagh was on edge, concern etched on her face.

Finally, I couldn't bear it any more. 'Oh, for fuck's sake, Clodagh,' I snapped, 'sit down. He'll be all right!'

Her eyes flashed and, without warning, she slapped me across the face. It was totally out of character for Clodagh, something she had never done before. It felt like a huge betrayal. I wasn't aware of it then, but that was a watershed moment in our relationship as sisters. We had been so close and mutually supportive, dealing with all sorts of turmoil, but no longer.

Of course, I look back now and see it was his influence. Clodagh was in his thrall. Alan was her all now, and she was in awe of him. He promised to look after her and provide her everything she clearly yearned for – security, stability and protection. He offered the safety and reliability she craved. Their relationship was intensely close from the beginning.

Despite the falling out, Clodagh asked me to be her bridesmaid when they got engaged not long after. I was thrilled to be asked and delighted for her too. I didn't care for Alan, but I knew he made her happy. They seemed perfectly matched – both level-headed and serious-minded. They shared a lot in common, including future careers in teaching.

The day came when Clodagh and I arranged to go shopping for the bridesmaid's dress. I was seventeen and had just started my first year studying auctioneering and valuations at the College of Further Studies in Ballsbridge. We arranged to meet in Jervis Street, and I had this feeling Alan would show up with Clodagh because she rarely went anywhere without him. Sure enough, I arrived at the appointed meeting spot and saw him waiting with her.

I was an incredibly body-conscious teenager, concealing my intermittent eating disorder. I was not prepared to get dressed and pose in outfits in front of a guy I hardly knew. I was adamant that Alan would not come dress-shopping with us.

'Okay, we'll see you later, Alan,' I said cheerily, hoping he'd take the hint.

'Oh, no, I'm coming too,' he replied.

I stared at him in amazement and turned to Clodagh on the busy shopping street. 'There's no way I'm trying on dresses in front of Alan.'

But Clodagh frowned, annoyed that I'd suggested Alan leave us. 'Why are you being difficult? Alan's here, and he's coming with us.'

I turned to Alan. 'I'm not trying on dresses in front of you. That's just not going to happen.'

'Well, it's my wedding too, and I want to be involved in all decisions.'

'Well, you don't decide what I wear,' I said.

I addressed Clodagh again. She was bristling with annoyance now, but I didn't care. 'Give me a call when you're ready to do this, just the two of us,' I said, turned on my heel and stalked off down Jervis Street.

I remember feeling furious. Why was a man insisting on coming dress-shopping? That was plain weird. And why was Clodagh allowing it when she could see how uncomfortable I was?

It was a battle I was never going to win. Clodagh got Mam involved in the row, and the pressure to conform piled on. I said I'd pick my own dress, but I wasn't allowed to have the one I wanted. Instead, I was brought to a dressmaker who put the measuring tape around me and remarked, 'Oh, you're a big girl, aren't you?' That was all I needed to hear to stop eating for months.

Clodagh was twenty-one, and Alan was twenty-two when they married on 12 July 2000. Their wedding day resulted in another rift between me and my sister. I got drunk, and Alan's parents were pin-wearing Pioneers, so Clodagh was furious with me. It was clear that I'd let the side down badly, and that put the final nail in the coffin of our relationship.

As soon as Clodagh left college, she and Alan moved to Navan. She taught at St Oliver's National School in the town, and he got a job at Skryne National School near Dunshaughlin.

They moved to Castlerahan after the birth of their second child, Niall, in 2004, and they remained there until the night of the murders twelve years later.

My life choices were different and far more chaotic. Whereas Clodagh sought security, my reaction to leaving home was wildness. Straight after college, I got work on Irish Ferries and had a ball – drinking, smoking and partying. I had boyfriends but never felt any desire to be tied down. I recently had to undergo garda vetting for a job and listed sixteen addresses in Dublin during those years.

When Alan and Clodagh had Liam, they asked Mam to be godmother. I let Clodagh know I was upset, but I don't think she realised how deeply she had wounded me. I got on with my own life, and didn't associate much with her and Alan. My relationship with them remained distant throughout the early years of their marriage. I breezed in and out every weekend, and whenever I spent time with Clodagh, Mam or Alan would be with us. Clodagh and I were never on our own.

Yet my sister was always there when I needed her. In my twenties, I was engaged, and the wedding was booked and planned for Oldcastle in Meath. I had been in the relationship for six years, but I got cold feet as the wedding date advanced. Everyone, apart from the groom-to-be, could see I was unhappy. I finally mustered the courage to cancel the wedding, but I was racked with guilt. My fiancé had done nothing to deserve the pain and humiliation of a broken engagement. Clodagh was a huge support during that time, assuring me again and again that I was doing the right thing.

But our relationship still had its limits. From early on, Clodagh had always made clear to me that 'If you tell me something, you tell Alan.' Alan had to be a party to everything we discussed. *Well, I sure as hell won't be telling you much, so*, I thought. Our relationship never developed into the intimate sisterly connection we should have had as adults. We started to regain that closer connection before she died, but that only came about with Clodagh's dawning realisation that her knight in shining armour was flawed after all. But she didn't see those chinks in his armour for a long time. Alan was her everything for many years.

While I was kept at arm's length, feeling like an outsider, Alan never managed to come between Clodagh and Mam.

Their relationship was forged in steel, and he must have realised he couldn't dent it. As a result, Mam was permitted into their tight family fold, and Alan always kept her onside. Even so, I recall Mam occasionally remarking how having time on her own with Clodagh was difficult. Anytime she and Clodagh went shopping, Alan would constantly call his wife, reminding her to buy things or asking where he could find something in the house. He was always present, even when he wasn't.

Mam lived with them for a short while between selling a house and buying another. She often tried to help around the house, and one day, she hung clothes out to dry. Later, she spotted Alan busy re-pegging and re-hanging the clothes fluttering on the washing line. When she cooked dinner for them, he lifted the lids, checked the water levels in the pots and insisted on covering the vegetables with more boiling water.

'Are you trying to drown them again, Alan?' she'd joke, but the inference was clear – she wasn't doing things to his exacting standards. She shrugged these incidents off as I did. It's Alan, and he has his peculiarities, his way of doing things. Anyway, isn't it great to see a man get involved in the housework?

But no one could fail to notice how much Alan influenced Clodagh. When Clodagh was pregnant for the third time, we sat around the dinner table one night, speculating whether she'd have a boy or a girl.

Clodagh was slicing into her roast beef when she added: 'Well, it's the male who decides the baby's sex.'

My brother Tadhg looked up, a twinkle in his eye. 'So, has Alan told you yet what you're having?' he deadpanned.

Everyone laughed because it was funny, even if it was gently mocking. We all knew Alan's word was gospel to Clodagh.

One year after my runaway bride drama, I met Richie and fell madly in love. It was a whirlwind romance, and everyone in my family fell in love with him too. Richie entered our lives as if he'd always been one of us.

By then, Tadhg was twenty-six, maturing into a beautiful blend of funny and caring. He was a beacon of light in my life. On bad days, I could pour my heart out to him, and somehow he'd always say or see something to lift my spirits. We laughed a lot together and fought like cat and dog. He was one of life's jokers, always seeing the fun and the ridiculous in things, especially in himself. I had drifted apart from Clodagh, but Tadhg and I remained close, and I loved being around him.

When I heard he was attending a Guns N' Roses concert at Dublin's O2 in September 2010, I invited him to stay overnight with Richie and me at our Kildare home. In Kill, it was closer to Dublin than the family home in Mountnugent. 'If you stay, we can drop you to Busáras in the morning on our way to work,' I suggested.

But Tadhg wouldn't hear of it. He said he'd stay with

us another time, and I didn't press him. Tadhg wasn't a big Guns N' Roses fan, but he received a free ticket to the show. That night, fans bottled the band four songs into their performance, prompting lead singer Axl Rose to walk off the stage. Tadhg was one of many who left early thinking the show was over, although the band returned to the stage an hour later.

And then I got a phone call at 2.20 a.m. that brought my world crashing down. The words almost strangled Mam as she uttered the unimaginable: Tadhg had returned home from Dublin after the concert and taken his own life. His death was completely unexpected and inexplicable. We lost Tadhg on Thursday, 2 September 2010, and I'd never known trauma or grief like it.

Even in my fog of grief, I saw that the tragedy came like a punch to Richie's gut too. Three months earlier, Richie and I had announced our engagement. Tadhg had been so happy for us and said he couldn't wait for our big day. Richie was aghast, staggered by what Tadhg had done. I remember how tightly we gripped each other in the days following my little brother's death. It was as if we feared letting go in case we lost each other.

'Why, Richie? Why would Tadhg do that?' I sobbed, but Richie couldn't answer me. Nobody could. Instead, we fervently promised each other that no matter how hard life got, neither of us would ever do that.

The devastation I felt after Tadhg's loss almost destroyed

me, and darkness descended for a long time. My mind churned with all the things I could have done and didn't. Why didn't I try harder to make him stay with us that night? Why didn't I argue more? I could have stopped this if I had just made him come to Kildare after the concert. Why didn't I talk to him more? I started punishing myself for not convincing him to stay and for not being a better sister. I stopped eating for months.

I hit out blindly at everyone. I wrote an unsent letter to Axl Rose, blaming him for not staying on stage. If only he had performed like he was supposed to, Tadhg wouldn't have returned home early, and Mam would have been there. If only. If, if, if … This is what grief does.

Much of what happened after my brother died is a blur, but I'll never forget that lonely journey in the ambulance with Tadhg, travelling from our home to Cavan general hospital. Usually, a hearse took a body to the mortuary, but out of respect for Mam, a valued nurse in Cavan General, we were given the privilege of accompanying Tadhg in an ambulance.

Somehow, though, even gazing at my brother that night, his death didn't seem real. Tadhg had had so many plans to travel, but that ambulance journey was our last trip together.

The only other thing I remember vividly was Mam saying, 'This is as bad as it gets.' She remembers saying that too. And I agreed. Mam's right. This is as bad as it gets.

5

Love

I first met Richie, the love of my life, on Monday, 19 January 2009. My hair was blonder than usual after a recent visit to the hairdresser, and my skin was darker thanks to a new spray tan. Together, they provided the confidence boost I needed for my first day as human resources administrator for St Vincent's private hospital in Dublin.

The HR executive offered to show me around the hospital and introduce me to everyone. We started on the ground floor, and she gestured this way and that.

'Now, if you go to your left down there, you'll get to the radiotherapy …'

But my eye was caught by a man strolling along the corridor towards us. Something about him struck me straight away. It helped that he was tall, dark and handsome, with a shock of dark curls and brown eyes. We exchanged a brief flicker of eye contact as he passed.

I barely managed to resist the temptation to turn and gaze at him as I heard his footsteps ascend a flight of stairs behind me. I could see the HR executive's lips move as she talked, but I was completely zoned out. I never heard a word she said.

Invisible threads seemed to draw us together because I would soon learn this man felt the same connection. Don't look back, he told himself. Don't let her see you looking back. Instead, he went straight to his supervisors, who knew everything that went on in the hospital. He noted my platinum blonde hair and spray-tanned skin and came to the wrong conclusion.

'Who's the new Swedish one in HR?' he asked the women.

'Who?'

'The new blonde.'

'She's from Cavan, ya dope!'

Meanwhile, my hospital tour continued, and the HR executive brought me to an office where I locked my gaze with that of the brown-eyed man again. He was introduced as Richie Connolly, and he and his colleague Keith, at the next desk, were catering officers.

Richie and I smiled at each other and made some small-talk, the extent of our contact that day.

The next day Richie sent me an email asking for the home address of one of the hospital employees. Surely he knows I can't hand him someone's details, I thought. But the request was only a pretext to make contact. One email led to another, and his emails went from work to personal very quickly. I started receiving these hilarious missives every day. You couldn't call them emails; they were more like essays, crazy snapshots of the interior life of Richie Connolly.

During these emails, he mentioned that he was looking for somewhere to live because he was moving out of his rented accommodation in Tallaght. He had left his girlfriend, but he didn't say so. Emails flew back and forth between us.

'I can see the steam rising out of that keyboard,' Keith would say, as Richie pecked away furiously. I rushed into work many mornings, hoping to find another essay waiting in my inbox. It took two weeks before he asked me out, and we went on our first date on 7 February 2009. I've never forgotten the date because it was also Tadhg's birthday.

Breaking with the convention of sharing the first kiss after the date, we kissed the minute we met in town that evening. We went to the Market Bar on Fade Street in Temple Bar for drinks and then for dinner in a nearby restaurant. I didn't care where I went; all that mattered was that I was with Richie. As the world swirled around us, we held fast, eyes locked and laughing. We had the best date ever. It was like we had known each other all our lives. I remember Richie laughing when I ordered a pasta dish.

'You're a fearless woman, Jacqueline Coll, ordering pasta on a first date.'

But something about Richie excited and calmed me at the same time. I didn't care about appearances when I was with him. I felt instantly at home.

We said, 'I love you,' quickly, and never stopped saying it. I lived in a rented apartment in Tallaght, and Richie (who'd recently moved back in with his parents in Clondalkin) would collect me for work every morning and bring me home every evening. By May, we were looking to buy a house together. We viewed places in Wicklow and Clane – anywhere we could afford within the commuter belt around Dublin. We found our new home in Kill, in Kildare, and moved in by November, less than nine months after our first date. I loved Kill because the area reminded me of Emmerdale and the Yorkshire Dales, and I was a huge soap fan.

Unfortunately, the soundproofing between the houses was so bad that you could hear the neighbours change their minds. For some incomprehensible reason, they bought a St Bernard puppy. It grew to the size of a horse and had a bark so loud it was like he was in the room with us. We used to joke that we lived next door to the Dingles, Emmerdale's famously loud and colourful family.

My love affair with TV soaps continued, and I watched them while Richie made dinner and cleaned. He treated me like a queen, and I shamelessly let him. I shouldn't have, but I did. I rarely even drove when I was with him because he chauffeured me everywhere and couldn't do enough for me. I was spoilt. And he did it all with a smile.

'I'm like a frog in a sock around you,' he said one day.

'A frog in a sock?'

'Jumping blindly around the place – overexcited.'

It was one of the many things he said that made me laugh. After that, my pet name for him was Kermie, Miss Piggy's endearment for Kermit the frog.

Richie pointed out that I'm not a morning person. We'd arrive at work together, and he'd be all chat, greeting everyone around us with a smile. I'd hear him heading off down the hospital corridor.

'Hi, ladies, how are you all this morning?'

I would roll my eyes, head for the sanctuary of my office and shut the door until I was on my second cup of coffee. I laugh now when I watch our child, Richie's carbon copy, dancing around the house at the crack of dawn. Richie was full of cheery energy, and everyone fell for his easy charm and warmth. His colleagues in the hospital loved him.

We didn't go out much after buying our house as finances were tight. Also, living in a commuter town rather than a community, we didn't know many people. That didn't matter to us because we loved spending time at home. Richie had two great pastimes, one of which was cooking, and I always knew what we were having for dinner by the ring of food around his feet. He'd leave a trail of destruction through the kitchen, but he was an excellent chef.

His other beloved pastime was golf, and he enjoyed a round most Saturdays with friends. I always joked that I was a golf widow, but now I flinch thinking of that phrase. My less frequent social excursions usually involved long, boozy lunches or dinners in Dublin with the girls. Richie always collected me afterwards, and inevitably, I'd tumble into his car, drunk on gin and the rush of emotion upon seeing him again. I've replayed the scene in my head and heard his laughter so many times.

'I jush love you soo mush, Risshy!'

'The state of you, Jacqueline Coll. You can't be let out anywhere!'

We never argued. On a rare occasion, if I took the hump over something he did or said, I could never be annoyed for long. He wouldn't take me seriously, merely bat his big brown eyes at me and say, 'G'wan, Jacqueline, gis a kiss!' How could you stay mad at someone like that? I felt so lucky to find a man like Richie, and so happy that he fell in love with me.

Many of our friends and colleagues were getting married around that time, and in May 2010, Richie and I attended four weddings and a funeral. (Richie's grandmother sadly died.) To Richie's great amusement, I caught the brides' bouquets at all four weddings.

On a sunny day the following month, I drove to Dundrum shopping centre to find something to wear for yet another hen night. Richie stayed home to clean the house and get a few things done. We usually did our own thing when we were apart, but this time, he texted me repeatedly to see where I was and how the shopping was going. It was sweltering as I drove home and I was stuck in traffic for ages, hot and frazzled when I pulled into the driveway. Richie flung open the front door, full of energy. *He's doing the frog in the sock thing again*, I thought.

'Hurry up! We're going on a picnic,' he announced.

'Give me a break, Richie. I'm sweating,' I said. 'Can we have the picnic in the garden? I don't want to get into the car again.'

'Where's your sense of adventure? We're going to Donadea Forest.'

I sighed to myself. Donadea was about twenty-five minutes from where we lived but, reluctantly, I got back into the car. Richie lost his way on the journey, and I remember laughing because he became so frantic about it. When we got to the forest, he unpacked a bag with champagne and gin, cheese and crackers – everything I love. We ate, drank, read the newspapers and basked in the sunshine. The midges rose as the sun went down, and I got distracted, swatting wildly around me with the newspaper and scratching myself.

That was when Richie chose to utter the words: 'Jacqueline, how would you like to be Mrs Connolly?'

I turned to see him on one knee with the ring in his hand. I wasn't sure if I heard him right. He had caught me completely off-guard, and you never knew with Richie.

'Is that real?' I asked.

'Of course, it's real,' he said, his tone indignant.

It took me a while to realise Richie was proposing to me. Eventually I flung myself upon him, kissing him madly as my answer.

While I'd been shopping in Dundrum, Richie had gone to Liffey Valley to collect the engagement ring. Then he had spent ages in the garden turning it this way and that to see the sparkle, wondering if he'd picked the right one. He needn't have worried. I loved it at first glance and I still wear it today on my right hand.

I was so happy about growing old with Richie and thought the laughter would never stop. Richie's parents once bought us a voucher for a weekend in Clare, and we ended up standing on the Cliffs of Moher on a rain-soaked, foggy day.

'If it's sunny, you can actually see the Statue of Liberty from here,' Richie announced.

I wasn't thinking. 'Really? That's amazing!'

He exploded with laughter. 'Oh, my God, Jacqueline,' he managed. 'The things you come out with. I can't believe you said that.'

I warned him if he told anyone what I'd said we were done!

When we went to my home in Clontyduffy, Richie usually headed for the kitchen, where he'd assemble cheese platters for Mam and me. I often went to bed, and Richie would stay up drinking and chatting with Mam half the night. As a future son-in-law, he was quite different from Alan Hawe.

He fitted so perfectly into my life that I soon couldn't remember a time before Richie. We tossed around ideas about where to get married but finally agreed that Clodagh's local church, St Mary's in Castlerahan, was the perfect choice. The picturesque old church is set on a hill, surrounded by trees and nature. The wedding day was set for Thursday, 8 December 2011.

We agreed to buy each other a wedding present. I got Richie measured for a new set of golf clubs, and he bought the treadmill I asked for. That didn't stop me teasing that he only bought it because he didn't want a fat bride. Tadhg had died the year before, and I was still in the throes of an eating disorder. I pounded away on that machine day after day, trying to exorcise my demons.

I was in a salon in Castlerahan for a hair trial before the wedding when I collapsed and started convulsing. I had never had a fit in my life.

Clodagh got me to Cavan general, and I spent a week in the hospital. At one stage, I was transferred to Monaghan where, under sedation, I proposed to the doctor in charge. 'If you marry me, you won't have to buy me a ring,' I told him, pointing at his ruby ring. 'You can give me your one.'

The ambulance returned me, still groggy, to Cavan general where Richie was anxiously waiting.

'Oh, Richie,' I wailed. 'I'm so sorry – I'm after proposing to a doctor!' He never let me forget that I'd proposed to another man weeks before our wedding.

They did every test – scans, ECGs, ultrasounds, a lumbar puncture, and explored a possible diagnosis of multiple sclerosis. In the end, they found nothing wrong with me. I was suffering from stress and grief and trying to run away from both on a treadmill.

As our wedding day arrived, Richie warned me not to leave him standing in the church. 'If you're more than fifteen minutes late, I'm heading,' he said. 'I'm telling you, I'm outta there! There'll be no one there when you get to the altar.'

Of course, everything went awry that morning. I wanted to go to the grave to see Tadhg. The makeup artist was late. Worst of all, Clodagh and I underestimated how long it would take to get into the wedding dress. It had lots of panels to be closed and laced.

'Hold it straight.'

'I am!'

'Well, it's gone crooked again. Next time, hold it straight!'

'I did hold it straight, but you're doing it all wrong.'

'Oh, God, we should have had a dress rehearsal! I don't know what you're laughing about, Jacqueline. You'll wear that dressing-gown up the aisle if we don't figure this out.'

Clodagh told everyone that getting me into the wedding dress was harder than any workout she'd ever done.

Meanwhile, I'd left my phone somewhere, and poor Richie was panicking in the church, trying to call me. I was oblivious, floating around in my happy bubble, the happiest ever bride-to-be. By the time I got to the altar, I was an hour late.

'I'm so sorry. I didn't do it on purpose,' were my first words to Richie on our wedding day, but I was already forgiven. He was delighted I was at the altar, and so was I. Even though it was December, a Red Admiral butterfly appeared and fluttered around us all during the ceremony. The sight of it brought tears to my eyes. I was reminded of the day the funeral director arrived after Tadhg died, and Mam and I watched a Red Admiral alight on his leg. Seeing the butterfly seemed like a wedding gift from another realm, an assurance from Tadhg that he was still among us.

It was such a happy day. Now it seems like I'm writing about a different world and an entirely different person. That day was like a whole lifetime ago, one filled with so much joy, promise and innocence.

6

Gone

It was a Friday night and, as usual, Richie and I were sitting in and watching *The Late Late Show*. He was also browsing on his laptop and scanning the Irish Jobs website. He had been headhunted months earlier and moved to another post in hospitality services. However, it wasn't what he'd hoped it would be, and he wasn't happy there.

'What about getting your old job back in St Vincent's?' I suggested. 'You enjoyed it there, and you know they'd have you back anytime.'

He shook his head. 'You never go back, Jacqueline,' he said. 'You never go back …'

We were sixteen months married at this stage, blissfully happy and expecting our first child. We had attended the twelve-week scan in Naas general hospital three days previously, and were assured everything was going well.

I felt blessed snuggling up to Richie on the couch that night. We had everything going for us. We had a happy marriage, a baby on the way, our own house, good jobs and career prospects. I had just started a new job with the Queally Group in Kildare. I was also studying part-time for a post-graduate diploma in human resources management at the National College of Ireland.

Richie had options. His skills were in demand, and if he stuck out his current job for a few more months, he could easily move company.

The following morning, neither of us had a lie-in. I had to go to college, and Richie was off to meet his brother for his Saturday-morning game of golf. He was in fantastic form, and I groaned as he danced around the bedroom floor. He was always too chirpy in the mornings.

'Any missed calls from Ryan Tubridy?' he asked while he was getting dressed.

We'd entered a competition on *The Late Late Show* to win €20,000 the night before. However, entrants had to answer a call to win, and we'd gone to bed before the show ended.

'No, how about you?'

'Me neither. We didn't miss that boat.'

With the pregnancy, I felt wrecked a lot of the time, so I put my feet up on the couch as Richie prepared to leave.

'You'd better get moving, Jacqueline, or you'll be late!' he said.

He got down to my level and leant in for a kiss before he left.

'I love you,' he said.

'I love you, too. See you later.'

I left the house shortly after he did and sent him a quick text when I got into the college: I'm here now. Love you.

We said 'I love you' all the time.

A text pinged back. I love you too. Enjoy your day.

I was in my happy bubble again now that I had a baby on the way. We'd reached the three-month milestone and had our first scan, so I began sharing the news with fellow students. I was so happy that I wanted to tell the world.

A few hours later, I sent Richie another text. When I didn't hear back, I didn't worry. He sometimes got held up on the golf course. The game could go on for hours. Later I glanced at my watch again and thought it odd that he hadn't replied. I sent him another text, then another. *He should be home by now*, I thought, but I was determined not to worry.

Weeks earlier I'd had a complete meltdown when I couldn't reach him. I'd raced home frantic with fear and found Richie's phone downstairs while he was upstairs, fast asleep. I'd been having panic attacks since the sudden loss of Tadhg.

I was doing my best to cope. The previous year, Richie and I had helped set up a Kildare Darkness into Light five-kilometre fundraiser for Pieta House and participated in memory of my brother. But ever since Tadhg had died, I'd been experiencing anxiety that I couldn't seem to shake. I was hyper-vigilant, always expecting the worst to happen. I'd imagine all sorts when people didn't answer their phone straight away.

After the last scare, Richie had promised he'd be more careful. He said he'd answer my calls or texts immediately and never leave me fretting again.

So, when lunchtime became 2 p.m. and there was still no answer, I started texting under the desk during the lecture. Would you please answer me, Richie? I'm worried. Please, please, answer me. There was no reply.

I desperately wanted to jump into the car and drive straight home to Kildare, but I had to resist the urge. The lecturer said she would impart crucial exam information that afternoon and warned us not to leave early.

I already felt at a disadvantage in the class because I was studying for a post-grad without having a primary degree. To get accepted onto the course, I'd had to submit a portfolio of prior learning for assessment. The college awarded me credit for years of working in HR, allowing me to skip the three- or four-year first-degree course.

It was difficult to concentrate that afternoon when my heart was beating faster and faster, and my anxiety levels were soaring. I kept texting Richie under the desk, and still, there was no answer.

The clock ticked on, and my phone lay silent. It turned

half past three, and then a quarter to four. That was when I gave in.

'I'm sorry, but I have to go,' I said, and fled.

I struggled, carrying a bundle of ten big textbooks, the maximum number I could take from the library. I remember flinging the books into the car's front passenger seat before running around to the driver's side. It was a new car, and I hadn't driven it very often. As soon as I started the engine, an alarm went off and incessant high-pitched beeps filled the vehicle. I didn't know what I had done wrong.

The urgent beeps grew more prolonged the further I drove. I was already at my wits' end worrying about Richie, and now I had the added fear that the car was about to blow up. Tears stung my eyes, and my heart pounded, but I continued to drive. Richie still had not replied, so I had to get home. (It was much later that I realised the weight of the books had triggered a sensor in the seat, and the alarm was merely urging the 'passenger' to use the seatbelt. I had no clue.) By the time I reached Newlands Cross on the outskirts of Dublin, the alarm had stopped.

I caught up with an ambulance on the way, and it was like a bad omen. I'd always heard it was unlucky to see the back of one, so I passed it. The stretch of road between Newlands Cross and Kill had a speed limit of 100 kph, and I remember looking at the speedometer as it reached 152 kph. I was also frantically dialling Richie and, still, there was no answer.

I had been trying him for hours now, and I was sick with a gnawing fear. I knew in my heart that something was seriously wrong. Had there been a crash? Maybe he was ill, had had a turn and collapsed in the house. Or perhaps he'd had an accident.

Everything raced through my head except the appalling scene I witnessed when I rushed through the front door of our house. I never for a millisecond thought that Richie would ever do what he had done to himself, me, us. We had promised each other in the wake of Tadhg's death that never, no matter what life threw at us, would we ever do what my little brother had done.

But Richie had broken that promise, and all I could do when I saw him was shriek, 'No!' again and again, as if the force of that denial could undo what had been done.

But it was true. I found the man I loved most in the world, the most vivid presence in my life, my best friend and my happiness, lifeless in our hallway on Saturday, 6 April 2013. The guards said afterwards that he had thirty-eight missed calls from me on his phone.

7

Acceptance

I must have told the emergency operator, 'I think he's dead,' because she was insistent. Cut him down. Help is on the way, but you must cut him down. Immediately. She made it sound imperative, and I must have felt a tiny flicker of hope because I rushed to do what she said. I used scissors from the set of knives in a wooden block on our kitchen counter.

It was a struggle because my husband was six foot two, but I held him in my arms and tried to breathe life through his lips. I tried CPR. I did everything they told me. It felt like a lifetime, but the paramedics arrived in six minutes and started work on him. I knew, though: I could see their faces were set in a grim line. They knew.

I thought of Clodagh and somehow remembered she was at a wedding in Navan. Location-wise, she was closest to me. I was free-falling into a vortex of darkness and needed someone to hold me. I centred myself and rang Alan Hawe, calm, sensible Alan.

'Richie is dead,' I said. 'You need to take Clodagh out of the room and tell her that. Tell her I must have her with me now. I need her now.'

Finding anyone after they have inflicted violence on themselves is horrifying, but it's even more horrendous when you love that person. The pain I felt was so unbearable that I thought I must be having a heart attack. I didn't care if I was. I would gladly have died then.

My hands trembled so severely when I called Mam that I couldn't get the phone to work. She said afterwards that she hardly recognised my voice. She could only hear what sounded like a distraught child at the end of the line. 'Richie's dead, Mam. Richie's dead!' Mam would have come too, but she had Clodagh's kids and was further away from me. It would take time.

The guards called a GP, and I stared at him in shock. I could hardly speak for sobbing, but I heard myself telling him, 'I'm pregnant.' I said it as if that should be a mitigating factor, and they should do something more to bring Richie back. I remember him shaking his head, and the eyes that met mine were weary and sad. 'There's nothing I can do,' he said. 'There's nothing anyone can do.'

At some stage in this horror, I found Richie's note. I scanned it anxiously, hoping this would somehow resolve everything, maybe even tell me it was all a terrible hoax. But his note was brief and held no answers. There was nothing to say why he was about to do something so desperate, so final.

Richie's family arrived and stood in the garden as the guards and the ambulance crew milled around. They were taking Richie's body away, and the guards wanted me to go with them to identify him formally at Naas general hospital. Richie's family didn't want to do it. That was when Clodagh arrived, and only for her, I would have had to do it on my own.

Within hours, the searing pain was replaced by numbness, detachment and cold, icy shock. Jesus Christ, Richie, you talked to me about everything. We did everything together. I'd thought there was nothing we didn't know about each other and nothing we couldn't work out together. How could you do this to us? Why didn't you let me help? Why?

Nothing made sense. Richie and I were hopeful and excited as we left our house on Wednesday for the first scan of our baby. Three days later, he left our home in a hearse.

I remember Gerry arriving at the house with Mam. 'This is all my fault,' I cried. They were my first words, and I believed them. I had this awful feeling that I had failed Richie in some terrible way. How had I not known that my husband was in such anguish that he would take his own life?

But Gerry grabbed me. 'Jackie, this is not your fault,' he said, almost shaking me. 'Sure, you loved him, and he loved you. How could it be your fault?'

God, I clung to those words, repeating them again and again, and they have helped me many times since, but they were hard to believe for a long time.

I'll never forget lying on the couch that night as a world of horror, one without Richie, spun around me. 'What am I going to do? Where am I going to bring Richie? How can I bury him here when we don't know anyone?'

Somehow I was already thinking about the future. I knew I didn't want to be in our house without Richie, but if I buried him in Kill, I would have to stay because I could never leave him there on his own. In the early hours of Sunday morning, it dawned on me. It's the place where we married, and no matter what happens, I'll always be going home . . .

'Maybe I could bury him in Castlerahan,' I told Mam. Looking back now, I don't know how I managed to work that out. I felt so grateful to Alan because he went to the local parish priest, Father Kelly, and arranged for the funeral to take place there.

Time became shapeless, and after that the days rolled into one another. The world seemed shrouded in a dark fog of shock and disbelief. Clodagh was worried about the baby and arranged another scan days after Richie's death. She brought me to the Hawe family GP, Dr Paula McKevitt, in Oldcastle. I remember the growing sense of horror as the doctor searched for a heartbeat on the Doppler ultrasound that day. She tried to reassure me that it was probably too early in the pregnancy for a scan to find a heartbeat. She arranged for another the day after Richie's funeral in the early-pregnancy unit at Cavan general hospital.

But I stumbled out of the surgery, distraught. 'Oh, God, Clodagh, now I've lost our baby!' I cried. I'd lost my husband, and now I was convinced the baby was gone too.

Richie's wake took place in Murphy's funeral home in Naas on the Tuesday after his death. We followed the hearse up the motorway to Cavan for the funeral the following morning, staring at the big spray of flowers on the coffin. Anytime I'm on that road now, I drive fast to avoid repeating the slow, deliberate journey, the vision of flowers.

That morning, I gazed at Richie's coffin before the altar, the same place where I had lit our wedding candle sixteen months earlier. It seemed as if I was trapped in some terrible nightmare I couldn't wake up from. On an icy cold Wednesday, 10 April, I saw the two priests who had married us help to lower the love of my life and father of our child into his grave.

I was on autopilot, doing what I was supposed to but not comprehending what was happening. I hardly recall anything in the days after Richie's death. The only thing I remember with clarity was the day after Richie's funeral when Mam brought me to Cavan general for my scan. It seemed like a miracle when it showed a steady heartbeat. Suddenly a shaft of light pierced the darkness, and I felt I had something to live for.

But my anxiety levels soared, and I fretted the whole way through the pregnancy. With every twitch, I felt certain I would lose the baby. Every time I had a scan, I cried with relief that everything was okay, but I lived in dread of the day that it wouldn't be.

In the weeks and months after the funeral, I spent much of the time driving up and down between Kildare and Cavan. I spent hours at Richie's graveside in Castlerahan, trying to make sense of what had happened. I cried so hard. Uncontrolled bouts of sobbing racked my body until my head ached, and the hard, painful lumps in my throat made it difficult to breathe.

When I wasn't at the grave, I was reading his note or trying to distract myself by studying for exams or submitting assignments. But I read that note every single day, asking, *Why, Richie? Why?* Butterflies, Red Admirals, appeared everywhere, like little messages of love and hope from beyond the grave. Maybe I was just looking for signs. Who knows?

But the predominant feelings I experienced in the early months were disbelief and terrible guilt. I stood there gazing down at the clay mound, thinking, *This is not real.* I couldn't accept that Richie was gone and that he would no longer be part of my life. I couldn't believe that this had happened. I kept expecting to hear his key in the door or his car pulling into the drive.

I blamed myself for not stopping him, for not getting home sooner, for not recognising his distress, for not seeing the depth of his pain. I felt like a failure. How did I miss it?

Others pointed accusing fingers at me too. Twelve years on, I still hear blame, and my husband's suicide has been used as a rod to beat me.

'You should have seen the signs,' one angry person told me, hurting me deeply. Those wounds heal eventually, but the scars never go away.

At Richie's wake, someone else said, 'You have to respect his decision to leave.' I stared at him, stunned. How the hell was I supposed to 'respect' that decision? And I don't know how often I've been told that I need to 'get over' Richie, like it's a switch I've failed to flick.

But the worst thing ever said to me took place at a large social gathering. 'Do you think,' a man near me asked, 'your husband killed himself because you didn't give him enough sex?' I don't know why he said this. He may have thought he was being funny or smart. I don't know. A woman who overheard him turned on him and verbally roasted him, and I was grateful for her support. But I walked out blinded with tears and took a taxi home, sobbing all the way. It wasn't only because it was a cruel and crude comment, there was that inference of blame, and it never fails to hit a nerve.

It has taken me years to accept what happened. Since then, remarks have been made and accusations hurled that have only served to re-traumatise me and prolong the process of acceptance. The flashbacks, the intrusive thoughts, the scents, the sight, and the trauma of what happened are never-ending. You can never forget it. I didn't know it for a long time, but

I have had post-traumatic stress disorder since that day, a condition I will suffer from for life. I can learn to cope better with the awful thoughts, but I will always have to live with the memories.

When Tadhg took his own life, no one blamed our family. But I didn't imagine the accusing eyes and comments after Richie died. Maybe there's misogyny at work when a woman's partner dies by his own hand. When there are no answers, it's easier to explain the death by laying it at the feet of the wife or girlfriend.

Of course, I also experienced great kindness from neighbours, friends and others. With the death of a partner, the financial strains can be enormous. When the death is by suicide, finances become even more complicated. Suddenly, I faced legal battles on every front and had to hire solicitors, which added to the costs.

After the probate was completed and the money was released to pay for Richie's funeral, I went to Murphy Brothers funeral directors in Naas. They were so kind and patient during and after the funeral that I was relieved to hand over a cheque to pay them and tick one more debt off my list. Murphy Brothers never lodged that cheque. It was a great kindness to a fragile, financially struggling widow with a newborn. I never expected it, but I have always deeply appreciated it.

I had only been working with the Queally Group in Kildare for six weeks when Richie died, and they couldn't have been kinder to me in the aftermath. I never returned to my job. I wasn't fit to work for a long time. But with a baby on the way, I knew I would have to provide for both of us, so I forced myself to continue studying for the post-grad. Losing myself in a stack of books each day distracted me for a while from the grief. Clodagh helped me study on many of those days.

I sat my employment-law exam a month after Richie died on Saturday, 11 May. That was also the day I felt our baby kick for the first time, which was a boost I badly needed. Our baby's little flutter reminded me that I had a purpose and had to keep going.

The morning of the exam, the Darkness into Light walk took place all over Ireland again. A year earlier, Richie and I had joined the suicide-prevention campaign in memory of Tadhg, and now Richie was gone too. My world had imploded, and there was no explanation for it.

For weeks and months, I searched the house for clues or evidence of something that could have driven him to it. He had never suffered from depression. I wondered whether I could have missed the signs. Could everyone have missed them? I didn't think so.

The day Richie took his life, he had been watching a war thriller called *The Hurt Locker* that he had recorded on Sky. I found the movie paused on the TV in the sitting room. I've never watched it. I couldn't bear to, but I remember asking the paramedics, and they assured me the issue of suicide did not arise in it. Richie also had papers, spreadsheets and documents from work spread around the couch. He must have come home after playing golf and started doing some work for the office. He wasn't happy in his job, but that wouldn't have triggered such a violent response. How do you go from playing a round of golf, working on spreadsheets and watching a movie to taking your life?

There had to be something more at work or somewhere else I didn't know about. My mind raced for months after he died. I felt there was nothing we didn't tell each other. Richie told me his deepest secrets – at least, I'd thought he did. But there had to have been an incident – something awful – he couldn't tell me about.

I've gone to the ends of the earth to find out the real reason he died, and I have failed. I believe somebody has a good idea of what happened and is not telling me. Whether it was something from his past or in his new job, somebody knows. I wholeheartedly believe that.

But Richie is the only one who can truly explain why he could no longer bear to live. So, I must come to terms with the fact I may never know the real reason. It has taken a long time, but I've also come to accept that taking his own life was Richie's choice. He decided to go. Just as Tadhg decided to go. They made that decision to end their lives for whatever deluded, misguided and mistaken reasons, but it was their choice.

My acceptance of Tadhg and Richie's decision only came after Alan Hawe had done what he did. Then I realised there's something even worse, even more cruel for survivors than finding a loved one dead by their own hand. Clodagh and her boys never chose to leave in the way Richie and Tadhg did. They never made that decision and were never given a choice. Alan Hawe took all their options from them on that August night.

8

Motherhood

Our baby was due on 14 October, according to the Coombe hospital in Dublin, and 21 October, according to Cavan general. Mam, Clodagh and I had lunch in the Riverfront Hotel in Virginia between my two due dates.

I was in two minds about the imminent birth. At one minute, I was excited about finally having our baby, and at the next, I thought, *How on earth am I going to have this baby on my own?* I never planned on being a sole parent. I was meant to do this with Richie. I felt very vulnerable.

I wanted to know the sex of our baby. I needed to plan, and I craved some certainties in my life. I didn't want any more shocks, surprises, bombshells or revelations. At eighteen weeks, the hospital scans revealed our baby's gender.

'Clodagh, you can clear your attic – it's a boy!' I said, and I remember how she whooped with delight. Clodagh had all her boys' baby garments stored in the attic, perfectly laundered, boxed and labelled, according to their size and age. I got all her boys' clothes until they died.

Mam and Clodagh couldn't fail to notice how huge I looked as we had lunch that day. Anytime I turned, it was like the moving bow of a ship, but there was still no sign of the baby budging.

'The midwives said I should try castor oil to bring on the labour,' I told them, grimacing. I had two lovely midwives, but I was appalled at their suggestion.

'It sounds like a good idea,' said Clodagh. She spent the rest of our lunch convincing me that I should jump-start the labour with castor oil. So that was why I found myself entering Lynch's pharmacy in Virginia shopping centre with Clodagh that afternoon.

Clodagh was by my side as I waddled to the counter, mortified. 'Can I have a bottle of castor oil, please?'

'Is it for yourself?' the assistant said, eyeing the giant bump.

'Yes,' I said, feeling hot colour flushing through my cheeks.

'Do you want the large bottle or the small one?'

When I turned to consult with Clodagh, I discovered I was alone. I spotted her slight figure at the far end of the pharmacy, bent over double, convulsing with laughter.

'The small one,' I said, in an even smaller voice.

I complained bitterly to Clodagh afterwards. 'I can't believe you left me alone up there.'

But Clodagh was still laughing too hard to care.

The months leading up to the birth were stressful. After the funeral, I was embroiled in a tangle of college studies, bureaucracy, paperwork and bills. The insurance company refused to pay out on the mortgage protection because Richie had taken his own life, so I faced a legal battle on that front.

According to the bank, I didn't even own the house. When we'd applied for the mortgage, the bank wouldn't accept my monthly rental payments as proof of my capacity to pay. The broker advised that Richie make the application and buy the house on his own, so even though I paid half the mortgage every month, my name wasn't on the deeds. We had been in our early thirties, and never even considered making a will, so Richie died intestate, meaning even more bureaucratic problems. (I'd implore anyone who is married to make a will to avoid the terrible headaches this can cause.) It was a mess, and I was sick with worry as well as grief. I didn't know where I stood and whether the baby and I would have a roof over our heads.

I remember the solicitor rang me, panicked on the day of Richie's inquest. 'What's the verdict?' she asked. 'I need to know. I'm in the High Court now.'

Eventually the insurance company paid up, and I finally got the house, but it was a long, stressful battle. Overnight, my life went from carefree and pampered to careworn and anxious. I had to take on the sole responsibility for everything, including our baby. Even the little things became traumatic. I remember trying to get the internet provider to change the account to my name. Every time I called, Customer Services insisted they needed to speak to the account holder. After my tenth attempt, I shouted down the phone: 'He's dead! He can't talk to you!' It's hard to believe, but these companies seemingly couldn't accept that people die.

Adding to the stress was my inability to decide where I wanted to be or what to do. After building a life with Richie, learning to live on my own was more complex and traumatic than I'd expected. When I was in Cavan near Richie's grave, I felt guilty for not being at our home in Kildare. When I was in our home in Kildare, I felt uneasy on my own. A chill ran through me every time I passed through the hall, and I was scared to turn my back on the spot where I'd found Richie. I didn't want to leave our home, but I didn't want to stay. I couldn't settle anywhere.

I spent much of my time in a kind of limbo. I kept driving to Richie's grave, where I could spend hours amid the serried rows of granite headstones. I still couldn't believe the man I'd loved, married and planned a child with was lying under the mound of clay before me. Richie was my best friend, and my future was mapped out with him. Now he was gone, and it seemed like my future was too. How am I going to live without you? I asked him constantly. I was crushed by the weight of sheer loneliness I felt. Only the thought of our baby kept me going.

After that lunch with Mam and Clodagh, I looked at my vast size in the mirror and decided it was time. I consumed thirty millilitres of castor oil in orange juice. Within hours, I was in labour at Cavan general hospital. However, many hours of grinding pain later, my baby showed no sign of arriving. As I had no threshold for pain, my labour was torturous for Mam and Clodagh.

'Oh, my God, it can't get any worse than this!' I cried out at one stage, and I was nearly sure I heard Clodagh snorting behind my back.

Later, much later, she admitted she had laughed. 'What could I say?' she said. 'You had no idea what was coming.'

And I didn't have a clue until Gary was born after twenty-one hours of labour, arriving a few minutes after midnight on Monday, 21 October. My mam and Clodagh witnessed his arrival and looked after him for the first couple of hours of his life. I had to be brought to the theatre afterwards, and didn't see him or hold him until he was two hours old.

Still, I'll never forget the instant that tiny stranger was handed to me because the reality of my new responsibility hit me like a hammer. Shit, I have a baby! I don't know anything about babies! How am I going to look after him by myself? I worried that my child had drawn the short straw with me as his mother.

In the late hours of the morning, Mam and Clodagh went home. The ward was dark and quiet, and I had Gary lying on my lap. I looked at this tiny little marvel that Richie and I had created, watching his fists flail and legs jerk.

I gazed at him with growing awe and amazement, stroking his plump cheeks and clenched fingers and admiring his tiny, perfect fingernails. I expected him to have Richie's big brown eyes, but he was born with my blue ones. I thought he was the most beautiful baby in the world.

It was just baby and me in our little world, and a sense of elation took over. The primal sense of protectiveness, love and possessiveness I felt for him was almost overwhelming. I took his first photo then as he slept. 'It's just you and me now, kid,' I whispered to him that morning, and that's the way it's been ever since.

His name had been decided nearly five months earlier – as soon as I learnt I was having a boy. Richie had picked the name the week before our first scan. We had started discussing baby names over a coffee in the Liffey Valley shopping centre in Clondalkin.

We agreed on a girl's name straight away. She would have been Mary Kate Connolly after my mam, Mary, and granny, Mary Kate.

Deciding on a boy's name turned out to be more contentious. 'I was thinking Oscar if it's a boy,' I said.

Richie gave a derisive snort. 'No way! Like Oscar Pistorius? He killed his girlfriend – we're not calling him Oscar!'

The South African runner had made headlines for months that year, so Richie had a point.

'Well, I was thinking of Conor too,' I said.

Richie gave a disinterested shrug.

'Well, what do you suggest, then?'

He had clearly thought about it because he was ready with his reply. 'If it's a boy, I'd like to call him Gary.'

I nearly spluttered into my coffee in response. 'Not a hope in hell!' I said. 'That's not a baby's name. Gary's a man's name!'

I couldn't imagine calling any baby Gary.

'Well, I like it,' said Richie. 'And it's my middle name. I always wanted to be called Gary.'

'Let's put it on the list, and we'll talk about it again,' I said, but in my head, the name was already binned.

There was only one Richie for me, and that's why I never considered calling our baby after his father. So when I discovered I was having a boy, I knew straight away he had to be named Gary.

It was Richie's choice, albeit one I'd never have agreed to if he had lived. But Richie's suggestion was right, and I love the name now. I haven't encountered a single other child with it, and it suits him because he's sometimes like a little old man. Gary is very much like Richie in his mannerisms. He's thoughtful and kind, like his father, and comes out with the funniest things.

'You're gas, Gary.'

'I'm not a fart, Mummy!'

Someone said to me recently that it must be hard being a sole parent, and raising a child on your own is difficult, but it's not hard work with Gary.

After a difficult start to 2024, I decided to take Gary on his first sun holiday abroad. I'd always travelled with companions before, so I made things straightforward by booking an all-inclusive package to Spain.

On the first night, we went to the restaurant for dinner, and I left Gary with his meal while I returned to the buffet to select mine. Upon returning, he announced, 'I've ordered the drinks.'

I said, 'What do you mean you've ordered the drinks?' He was ten.

'Well,' he said, 'I ordered Fanta Orange for myself, water for the table, and I picked a Rioja for you,' pointing to the wine list.

He's like his father, always messing, so I assumed he was joking.

Moments later, a waitress appeared carrying a tray with not just a glass, but an entire bottle of wine.

In that instant, I saw his father's mischievous spirit shine through. *You are the cut of your dad*, I thought. I couldn't stop laughing, and the struggles of previous months were consigned to a distant memory where they belonged. We had a ball together.

For the first forty-eight hours after Gary was born, I felt

euphoric. I was like Supermam, ready to take on everything for my baby. Unfortunately, the high soon plummeted, and I started a slow descent into the depths of despair.

It started the day I brought Gary home from the hospital, and we went to stay in Mam's house for a few days. Realisation struck me: This is not the way things should be. This is not the plan. I should be in Kildare with Richie. It was all downhill after that. It was as if my body had kept me primed and fit to deliver the baby safely, then called it quits overnight.

Nothing could have prepared me for the intense hopelessness and darkness that hit me as I sank into the most terrible post-natal depression. What's the point of living without Richie? I thought. I've done my job and brought Gary here safe and sound. Maybe I can go now too.

A new mum dreams of being happy and smiling as she cradles her sleeping cherub baby. But all I wanted to do was die and be with Richie. Hormones and grief are not a good combination, and I very nearly didn't survive that first year. I felt hugely guilty that I couldn't be the mother our baby deserved and was so low at times that I thought Gary would be better off without me.

I went out somewhere one day, leaving Gary with Mam. I also left my phone behind, accidentally. I'd never done that before, so everyone was in a terrible flap when I returned. I don't know how long I was gone, but I remember Alan berating me when I got back. 'How could you be so inconsiderate?' he said.

In the end, I did what anyone does when the shit hits the fan. I dug deep and kept going. It's hard work, but I'd seen my mother doing it after Tadhg died, and I knew what to do. I forced a smile on my face and put one foot in front of the other.

The former CEO of Pieta House, Joan Freeman, organised counselling for me when I asked. Many times, all I did for the entire session was cry. I felt such pain that I couldn't form any thoughts or words.

But I went through the motions and kept going, even though some days felt like a lifetime. I attended my graduation with Gary when he was four weeks old and was presented with the President's Award for achievement at the college. I got through that unbearable second wedding anniversary by celebrating Gary's christening that day. I got through that first Christmas without Richie by taking it one day at a time. I had the support of Mam, Clodagh and Dr McKevitt but I refused medication. No matter how bad I got, I was Gary's sole carer and didn't want to be sedated or drugged. I wanted to be present for our baby.

Piece by piece, day by day, I started to emerge out of the darkness again. It took a long time, but my moods became more stable, the spaces between the terrible lows widened, and I started to feel stronger.

Mam sold the family home in Mountnugent and moved to Virginia. When Gary was eleven months old, I sold our home in Kill and moved into Mam's new house for a year.

I was constantly aware that my life wasn't meant to be like that. *How did I get here?* I kept asking myself.

It was all very strange. Only Mam and Clodagh had known Richie and were aware of my other life in Kildare. No one else did, so no one talked about him. No one really talks about him even to this day. People not really knowing my previous life is freeing, but sometimes it makes me feel very much alone. And even after all these years, I can still be overwhelmed by grief and loneliness for Richie.

On 8 December 2021 I dropped Gary at school, and as soon as I got back into the car, I put my head on the wheel and sobbed for twenty minutes. No one saw me. I was crying because it was our tenth wedding anniversary. I have all these memories that few around me share.

I have never felt angry with Richie for doing what he did, even though I could never understand why he did it. I was devastated that he didn't let me try to help him. And I'll admit I feel bouts of self-pity sometimes. When times are hard, I can get frustrated because I'm dealing with everything on my own. But I tell myself, I'm a big girl, I've come a long way and can stand on my own two feet.

Everyone rallies around Gary in Virginia. He is protected and looked after in the town. He's lucky to have Gerry as a male role model. Gerry takes him swimming, farming and to the hunt on St Stephen's Day. He takes him on the tractor down the fields and does all those male bonding things with him.

But Gary still finds it difficult sometimes not having a dad. He asks questions, and I answer them as honestly as I can in an age-appropriate way. I'm afraid I'll say the wrong thing, so that's where my psychologist, Dr Paul Gaffney, is invaluable. I call him for advice when I'm unsure how to respond to Gary's questions. When I see Richie's absence or his decisions affecting Gary, it's only then that I feel furious with my late husband.

Adjusting to this new life, in which Richie doesn't exist and never will, has been a long and difficult struggle. Yet I know Richie would be so proud of us – his beautiful, kind and caring son and a wife who swapped her nightly TV soaps for motherhood and a successful, busy career.

The loneliness has been overwhelming at times. Yet every time I see Gary's smile, I feel so grateful. It reminds me of how precious life is and, sadly, how much Richie is missing.

9

Aftermath

The same strange sense of numbness and disbelief I had experienced after Richie died came over me again in the days after Clodagh and the boys were murdered. I felt an even greater sense of unreality this time because of the isolation. The silence was almost too loud in the house. Few people came near us, and the media had descended on the area, so we didn't even go to the shops. I scrolled comments on Facebook, but we switched off the TV and the radio and avoided newspapers after the shock of reading about the brutality of Clodagh's death. It was too upsetting.

I rang our family liaison officer immediately after reading that report. 'Please tell me he didn't kill her with a hatchet,' I begged.

The officer said he had to speak with the investigation team, but he eventually confirmed the reports were accurate.

I was stunned. How could it be true? Alan loved Clodagh! I was appalled that I had to hear this information via the media. I look back now, and I think the horror was too overwhelming to absorb. Neither Mam nor I could process it. We couldn't reconcile that brutal, savage act with the man we thought we knew, the man Clodagh loved. God almighty, I remember even writing a tribute to Alan Hawe and defending him on Facebook in the immediate days after the murders.

Mostly, we sat in heavy silence. Mam and I, Carmel, Gerry and my cousins, Melissa, Audrey and Eileen, waited for news from the guards. We didn't know what was going on or when the bodies would be released. I remember feeling a deep longing to go to Richie's grave, but St Mary's Church and the cemetery are directly across the road from the school where Alan Hawe had been vice-principal and Niall and Ryan were pupils. The media were camped outside Castlerahan school that week, so I stayed away from the graveyard. I remained in the silence, waiting.

When I think back to those awful first days, it was such a lonely time. Mam and I didn't manage to make contact with the Hawe family for days after the murders. It didn't seem right to make arrangements for Alan's remains when his family might have other ideas. However, the parish priest, Father Kelly, rang, saying the bishop was anxious to settle arrangements for the funerals. By late on Tuesday, we felt we should be doing something, so I called the funeral director, Declan Finnegan, in Cavan.

Declan had handled my brother Tadhg's funeral and helped arrange a gravestone for Richie. He came to my house that night, and we started organising a mass funeral. Mam and I were still in shock, living in a surreal bubble and disconnected from reality. We expected the bodies to be released from Our Lady of Lourdes hospital in Drogheda to the undertakers on Wednesday. Father Kelly said he wanted the wake to take place on Thursday. We thought it was too soon and too rushed, especially if they delayed releasing the bodies. We hadn't even met with the gardaí at that point, so we didn't know what we were meant to be doing.

Finally, we got word that the guards would brief the families on Wednesday afternoon. Alan Hawe's parents agreed to attend that briefing, so it would be our first time speaking with them since the bodies were discovered. We'd met Alan's parents, Stephen and Olive, several times when they visited Alan, Clodagh and their grandchildren. Like most daughters-in-law, Clodagh was always anxious to make a good impression. She would almost sterilise the house before they arrived and, in the early years, warned Tadhg and me to behave and not swear in front of them. I remembered how she dressed the kids in clothes the Hawes had sent as birthday gifts, and everyone was ordered to be on their best behaviour. She was always thinking of their feelings.

Early on the morning of the garda briefing, Mam and I drove the familiar back road to Carmel and Gerry's house. We'd been doing so every day to avoid the media calling to the door. Stephen, Olive and her brother pulled up at Carmel and Gerry's just before the guards were due to turn up.

Mam and I hugged them in welcome, relieved to see them after the isolating ordeal we'd been through. We had been living in a vacuum for three days. If there had been a normal death in the family, we would have been surrounded by friends and neighbours. But people were not interacting with us. Maybe they didn't know how or thought we were surrounded by investigating gardaí. If anyone understood what we were going through, we thought it would be the Hawes. We were two families in crisis and in the dark about what had happened to our loved ones.

There wasn't a lot said. Mam related all that she knew from Clodagh about Alan's problems in school. The Hawes listened, and I remember thinking they were very calm and composed.

Three guards from the investigation team at Bailieborough garda station arrived soon after. The lead detective, a female garda and our family liaison officer offered their sympathies and filed into my aunt and uncle's sitting room.

I remember sitting there anxiously, waiting for everything to be explained to us, for everything to make sense at last. The detective opened his notebook and began to fill us in on the investigation so far. He said the forensics team was still working in the house, and then he dropped a bombshell.

'He left a note,' the detective said.

I was shocked. A letter didn't fit in with how I'd tried to explain everything in my head – Alan had gone mad and killed everyone in a frenzy, including himself.

'It was addressed "For family only",' the detective said.

'What does it say? Can we read it?' I think Mam asked that.

'I'm sorry. It's part of the investigation, but I've taken a few notes from it and I'll read them to you.'

The detective said Alan Hawe addressed his letter, 'To Mom, Dad, Mary [Mam], PJ, Enda [his two brothers] and Jacqueline.'

He read out the line that said, 'I am sorry for how I murdered them all, but I simply had no other way.' I remember him reading another line from the letter that said, 'Please cremate me and bury me at sea. Do not bury me as a Catholic.'

Unfortunately, the officer didn't read the part that said, 'Do not bury me with family.' We wouldn't hear that part of Alan Hawe's murder letter until much later.

I rolled the words over in my head, 'bury me at sea'. I remember thinking, *That's stupid. Why would we do that?*

Mam blinked on hearing those words too. 'Well, should we change the funeral arrangements?'

'No,' said the detective.

The Hawes said nothing at all.

The detective continued: 'His note also says, "Please get Clodagh's jewellery on the bed and give it to Mary."' I saw Mam flinch.

The detective added that the note also had instructions for his brother. 'Tell PJ to sell the car jeep.'

I immediately thought of Alan Hawe polishing his silver Kia Sportage every Sunday until it sparkled.

That was about all the three guards had to tell us that day. However, in the general hubbub of conversation as they were leaving, I heard one say to Mam that the school was mentioned several times in Hawe's letter. He said he believed whatever happened at the school was 'the catalyst' for everything that had taken place days earlier. The catalyst. I overheard those words myself. I understood it to mean that the school was at the centre of the investigation.

That night, I reimagined the crime scene and pictured Alan Hawe scribbling a few hurried lines at the kitchen table before he killed himself. I still never dreamed that he had written a five-page letter after he murdered Clodagh, Liam, Niall and Ryan. Or that he wrote more on the front and back of the envelope and left another loose sheet with a list of 'instructions'.

Those few lines read by the detective were all that were revealed to us for a long time. The guards gave us innocuous details, nothing that offered any insight into what had happened or why. We hadn't a clue. The media knew more than we did, but we had stopped reading or listening to the news after seeing the report that Hawe had used a hatchet to kill Clodagh.

We knew the bodies were about to be released to the undertaker, so we confirmed with the Hawes that the wake would take place on Friday, 2 September. The Hawes returned straight after to Kilkenny, leaving the funeral arrangements to Mam and me.

'We'll be happy with whatever you decide,' they said.

The timing was awful, as that Friday coincided with the sixth anniversary of our brother's death. We had to cancel Tadhg's anniversary mass scheduled for that day at Ballinacree Church in Meath. When Father Kelly came to the house for the first time on Thursday, we discovered the timing for the funerals on Saturday wasn't ideal either. A wedding was scheduled that morning, so the funeral mass couldn't start until 4 p.m.

I don't know why everything had to be rushed, but Father Kelly insisted on us finalising all the arrangements, explaining he was under pressure from the bishop. I began organising the details of the funerals. The first thing was to go to Clodagh's house to collect clothes for the undertaker and find some of the boys' possessions. We wanted to place a few beloved items with them in their coffins before they went to their eternal rest.

The boys. It was impossible to think they were gone. I couldn't imagine going into that house without hearing their laughter or seeing Ryan tear around on his little bicycle.

Their eldest, Liam, age fourteen, had grown so tall, sprouting up over the summer. He was just about to start back at Virginia College, entering his Junior Cert year. He was athletic and an enthusiastic member of Eagles Basketball Club and other sports teams but also studious, like his mother. He was ambitious and driven, always top of the class. He wanted to be the best at everything, and when he wasn't, it annoyed him. But he was warm and loving, and even though he'd reached those awkward teenage years, he was never too embarrassed to hug any of us.

Liam was responsible, too – a side of his personality that I wasn't so fond of when it got me into trouble. He told Clodagh he'd seen me texting on my phone in the car. (I maintained it was at traffic lights, but he said otherwise.) When he was younger, he and Niall loved to watch my makeup routine on a night out. They'd sit on the bed, mesmerised and horrified at the potions and warpaint being applied. 'But why do you want to make your eyes look black?' Liam asked, his face a portrait of confusion.

And he certainly didn't bolster my self-esteem before a night out. 'What's that shadow in the middle of your hair?' he asked another time, pointing at my dark roots.

That summer, our relationship began to evolve, and I could talk to him in a way that I couldn't with his brothers. I'd been able to tease him because he was starting to show an interest in girls. We also shared some of the same tastes in music, such as Avicii and Swedish House Mafia. Hearing the song, 'Don't You Worry Child', on the radio still brings a lump to my throat. At times, I hear it and think he's sending a little reminder that he's looking after us. Other times, I have to switch it off. I can't deal with the rush of emotion the words bring.

Liam was popular and had a wide circle of friends, boys and girls. He wasn't dating anyone, but one of his friends has since tattooed his initials on the inside of her arm on the spot 'nearest her heart'. Others continue to leave cards on his grave on his birthday and at Christmas. He was young, but Liam had already managed to touch people deeply. He was growing into a young man whom any parent would be proud of.

A week after their eighth anniversary last year, I met one of Liam's female friends from school. She has gone through college and is starting her career. She fondly recalled how they took class notes for each other and looked out for each other. I cried knowing Liam is still remembered and holds a special place in his friends' hearts.

Niall, the middle child, was eleven. He was my godchild and the sensitive, creative one in the family. He was quiet compared to the others, drifting about, doing his own thing. You'd hardly know he was there. He was obsessed with Lego and would lose himself in his creations, displaying the best ones on a shelf in the playroom. He had been so happy when he won a trip to Legoland Windsor Resort in England in the local GAA raffle that year. It was a trip he'd never go on. My friend Sinéad and I brought Gary to Legoland in England in 2021, and I thought of Niall and how he would have been in awe of the place.

Niall was an avid reader, too. He was short-sighted, so he always wore glasses. He was often engrossed in his Horrid Henry books or any by David Walliams. He loved reading the fart-and-poo lines from Gangsta Granny to his own granny. '"As she took each step, a little bubble of wind puffed out of her saggy bottom,"' he'd read aloud, shrieking with laughter.

Niall loved to bake. His favourite TV show was *The Great British Bake Off* with Mary Berry. He decided that when he grew up he would be a baker and open a shop in Virginia. His signature dish was chocolate brownies, but he also made lemon drizzle cake and iced buns, and was forever offering around trays of goodies. And there was no avoiding those calories because he'd be very offended if you didn't eat them.

Then there was little Ryan, the baby of the family, aged six. Ryan was a special baby from the start because he was the child Clodagh never thought she'd have. Doctors had told her she wouldn't have any more after Niall. Ryan was a real little imp, a tearaway, and seemed destined to be the life and soul of every party. I called him 'Ryan the Rebel' and I can still see him pedalling his bike furiously around the house, wearing his helmet with spikes on top of it like a little Sid Vicious. He made me laugh so much. 'Good luck with him!' I used to say to Clodagh. He was such a tiny little fellow, really slight and hugely affectionate, a child who would run to anyone for a hug. He looked up to his older brothers, so he shared Niall's passion for Lego. The three were so different, but all of them were sweet and gorgeous boys and so mannerly. Everyone who knew them loved them.

Clodagh only wanted the best for her children. She loved them all dearly, but they never got away with nonsense. She found sweet wrappers in Liam's school trousers and was furious that he'd been buying junk food. I remember the uproar when Liam denied it. But she was never as strict as Alan was. The boys would always scramble to attention when he was around. If they didn't respond fast enough, I remember his caustic tone as he drawled, 'Am I speaking in a foreign language?'

I dreaded entering Clodagh's house before the funerals, but I had their outfits to assemble and a list of things to gather as offertory gifts. I drove over to the house but sat in my car outside, taking deep breaths, trying to steady myself. Two gardaí had agreed to meet me at the scene, but I did not want to go in. Don't think about it now, was my mantra. Don't think about what happened. Get in, get their stuff, and get out.

Approaching the back door, I faltered: I saw pairs of shoes lined up outside – Alan Hawe's runners and shoes. Had he left them there or the gardaí?

Closer to the door, I saw traces of the Sellotape Alan Hawe had used to hang his warning note on the glass. I took another breath and entered the kitchen. I saw the table and remembered the last day I'd sat there with Clodagh. We'd laughed and cried about Tadhg and his pending anniversary.

My eye fell on the family lunchboxes laid out on the table: fruit already in them for the lunches Clodagh had planned to finish on Monday morning. Evidence of their everyday lives was all around me. A lump formed in my throat. I had to concentrate on the job I had to do. Let's go, Jacqueline, keep going. I picked up a framed photo of Ryan. He had made the frame in school and adorned it with fake gemstones. I keep it in my kitchen press. Sometimes, the picture stops me in my tracks, and I take it out. His cute little face smiling at me brings me to tears.

I headed for the playroom to pack a few of Niall and Ryan's Lego creations. The room was silent. Their toys and favourite games were still scattered around as if awaiting the boys' return. The emotions that rose in me were overwhelming – fear, confusion, despair – but I still couldn't accept the reality of what had happened. I was in shock, detached, disbelieving. *Don't think. Don't think about it now.* I retreated from the room with the Lego and headed for the sitting room.

I spotted Liam's most treasured possession – his new PlayStation PS4. His parents had promised that if he did well in his second-year summer exams, they would buy him a PS4. He was so happy when they gave it to him that summer, and now I was gathering it into a bag for his coffin.

I hurried on. The sooner I was finished, the sooner I could leave. I headed upstairs for Liam and Niall's room to get their clothes, but a guard stopped me on the landing.

'We're going to have to prepare you, Jacqueline,' he said. 'The boys' room is not fully cleaned. There are stains on the walls and beds that couldn't be removed.'

I had to keep going.

'I won't look at anything,' I assured the guard. And I meant it. I was determined to put my head down and head straight for the wardrobe to get their clothes. He just nodded and let me in.

But I couldn't miss it. A bloodstain splashed the length of the bedroom wall. The room swam around me as I stumbled towards the wardrobe. I screwed my eyes shut, but for an instant I was afraid I might vomit. I couldn't figure out who owned what. Don't think. Clothes. Concentrate on their clothes. I fumbled and cried and fumbled some more in their wardrobe. Oh, Jesus, is this Niall's or Liam's?

I tried to pull outfits together with matching pairs of shoes. It seemed like a Herculean task when all I wanted was to get out of that room.

I found a basketball for Liam and gathered some of his and Niall's favourite hoodies and trousers. I collected a trophy that Niall had won at basketball. I staggered out of the room, my face buried in a towering bundle of clothes, shoes and other possessions in my arms.

I carried them downstairs and took a deep breath. Ryan's

room next. I went back upstairs, glanced around the room and realised Ryan's mattress had vanished. The luminous stars he stuck to the top of his bed remained. He loved them because they glowed in the dark. I peeled one off and brought it with me. I've kept it safe for you, Ryan. I'll keep it safe for ever.

I kept looking for Ryan's favourite little white and brown bear, Dreamy. I knew it had to be there because Ryan would never have gone to bed without it. One of the guards hesitantly explained that it 'couldn't be salvaged'. He meant it was covered with too much of Ryan's blood. (Mam eventually found a replica of Dreamy, now in a glass jar on his grave.) I headed for Ryan's wardrobe, eyes down, blinkered against any further evidence of savagery.

When I finished with the boys' outfits, I searched for a dress for Clodagh. I knew the one I wanted – she'd worn it to Alan's brother's wedding the year before she died. I took, also, the photo of Clodagh posing with all her family. It's the family photo everyone is familiar with now because we released it to the media early in the investigation.

'It's better to approve one and send it out,' the guards said. 'Every time this story comes up, or there's another murder-suicide, the photo you give to the media will be the one they'll use. It's better to have them use one you like rather than the one they'll find instead.' They were right.

As I learnt more about the killings, though, I learnt to hate that photo. Alan Hawe stands at the extreme left of the picture. Even though he's at the edge, he's still a dominating presence, towering over his family. He's wearing a black wedding waistcoat over his white dress shirt and a silver tie in a Windsor knot. His spine is erect, his chest puffed, and his face wears a proprietary beam of pride. I see self-satisfaction and smugness oozing out of his every pore.

Clodagh is next, gentle and smiling. She looks lovely, her hands gracefully clasped in front of her lacy dress. Then there's Liam, glowing with warmth and kindness, in his blue shirt, almost as tall as Clodagh. (He soon outgrew her.) Further down the row is Niall, with his toothy smile and spectacles, shy but brimming with intelligence. Last, well below his shoulder, peeping into the photo, there is the wide-eyed, mischievous little Ryan.

Alan Hawe's ominous presence ruined that beautiful photo of Clodagh and the boys for me. We sent out another, a lovely one of Clodagh, Liam, Niall and Ryan. It doesn't include their murderer, and I wish the media would use it instead.

I tore through Clodagh's wardrobes for the peach dress she'd worn to that wedding but couldn't find it. I was shaken and flustered, though: maybe I just couldn't see it.

I described it to one of the guards, and he spotted it in a spare closet in another room. The odd thing was that the matching shoes Clodagh had worn with the dress were on her bedroom floor, in front of her wardrobe. They were dressy shoes, not the kind Clodagh would ever wear to school.

Also she was incredibly ordered and neat: everything had its place. She would never have left a pair of high heels out. I wondered if Alan Hawe had thought of everything.

It was the same with the jewellery he instructed should go to Mam. The jewellery boxes were left in a precise line along the bottom of his and Clodagh's bed. He even left a bag in which to pack everything. I glanced towards Clodagh's dresser and saw a gold watch Mam had given her, so I took that too. God help me, I even assembled an outfit for Alan Hawe that day but I forgot to bring his shoes. He went into his grave barefoot.

I was so relieved to escape the house and sank into my car. My fingers trembled as I turned the keys in the ignition. I headed straight for Lakelands funeral home in Cavan town, my heart thrumming in my chest.

On the way, I had to stop for fuel at the Applegreen petrol station in the village of Poles. As I went to pay, I saw the magazine stand stacked with bundles of the daily newspapers. All my family's faces, Clodagh and her boys, were plastered across every front page.

In that garage nobody knew who I was. But they must have wondered why the strange woman at the till was blindly rummaging through her handbag while tears rolled unchecked down her cheeks.

1 0

Last Visit

The last time I saw Clodagh was ten days before she and the boys were murdered. I had an appointment for Gary with the doctor on Friday, 19 August. Afterwards I thought I'd ring Clodagh and ask if it was okay to call over. I never made any impromptu visits to her house. That had become the unspoken arrangement between us over the years. If Alan answered the phone, I'd raise my eyes to heaven and make polite small-talk. 'How's your mother and father?' 'How are the boys?' All the while, I waited for the right moment to say, 'Can I speak to Clodagh?'

I often tried to meet Clodagh outside the house. I'd invite her for a coffee, but she'd say, 'I'll have to ask Alan and see what his plans are.' That would be the last I'd hear about coffee. If I wanted to see Clodagh and my nephews, I had to go to their house. And that meant seeing Alan, too, because he was always hovering. Clodagh and I would be in conversation, and he would just stand leaning in the doorway, arms folded, sometimes not saying a word. But he was there, this overbearing, silent presence. On other occasions, he'd be in and out of the room looking for things, asking Clodagh to get stuff for him. His actions always let us know that he was there.

He often stopped us mid-conversation to say, 'What's that now?' I'd mentally roll my eyes while Clodagh or I would have to repeat the entire conversation to him. He'd have to hear everything.

Mostly, I didn't like being around him because he made me feel bad about myself. I always felt as if I had to be on my best behaviour with Alan. He had this superior air about him, and he was always watching, waiting to pounce and voice his disapproval in myriad small ways. He might snort with derision or sigh with exasperation when I was talking. Or he'd let out a sharp 'Tsk!' in disdainful commentary on something I'd said. It rattled me. I always felt I had to be careful what I said around him. Clodagh appeared deaf to this, but when I was around Alan Hawe, I saw his pursed lips and scowls and felt inept. I believed he thought me stupid, but I know different now.

I remember relating a silly incident at work to Clodagh. A staff member in Clontarf Hospital was a big fan of Mickey Mouse and anything to do with Disney. She said she even had a Disney-themed Christmas tree. I laughed. 'So, basically, you have a tree covered with Mickeys,' I said. That's just my sense of humour. Things come out before I even think about them. Clodagh burst into peals of laughter when I told her the story. The woman in Clontarf Hospital thought it was hilarious too. Clodagh and I were still spluttering about the tree full of Mickeys while Alan was listening and watching.

'That's not funny,' he said, with a stone face, and it was as if he'd thrown a bucket of cold water over us. He wasn't part of the conversation but had to let us know he disapproved of my story. That was the way he was. He couldn't be silly for a minute.

Richie wasn't long passed, and Gary was a baby when Mam sold the house in Mountnugent and moved in with them for a brief time. I was alone in Kill, raising a newborn baby on my own. I remember asking to stay at Clodagh's house for the weekend.

'I'll have to ask Alan,' she replied. I was stunned. I couldn't believe she needed permission from him for her newly widowed sister to stay. I know now it wasn't her talking. Yet I couldn't say anything. I already felt like an outsider, hovering on the fringes of their family. In the back of my mind, I worried that they might close the door on me, that Gary and I might never see Liam, Niall and Ryan again. It was important to me to keep that connection, but it was difficult to hold my tongue.

On New Year's Eve 2015, I rushed home from Clontarf Hospital to pick up Gary. I booted it down the motorway avoiding memories of flowers. Apparently, I passed Alan as he drove Clodagh and the boys back from his home in Kilkenny. A half-hour later, I met Clodagh in SuperValu.

'You passed us on the motorway,' she said.

'I did?'

'Little wonder you didn't see us with the speed you were going.'

It all blew up from there, and suddenly I was banned from having the boys in my car again. This was Alan in Clodagh's ear. I rarely got to spend time with the boys on my own anyway, and I wasn't allowed to babysit them.

I wasn't the only one who had restricted access to the kids.

Carmel and Gerry asked to take Ryan out for an afternoon not long before he was murdered. Ryan was delighted to be invited because he loved being with his 'Granddad Gerry', It was all arranged. Carmel and Gerry brought Ryan back to their house with plans to bring him for a walk and stop for ice creams and lemonade. But they never had the chance. Forty-five minutes later, Alan turned up at their door to collect Ryan. It was bizarre, but we all shrugged.

'That's Alan for you,' we said.

A month after Richie died, I sat my post-grad exams and passed. A lot of my success was down to Clodagh. She had helped me study during those difficult weeks, drilling acronyms into my head so I could memorise the coursework. Of course, I wanted her at my graduation, but Alan put the kibosh on that too.

'I can't come,' she said. 'It means taking a day off, and Alan says we should keep our holidays in case any of the boys get sick.'

That hurt me. It was only one day, and it was my first graduation ceremony. It had been a monumental struggle to sit those exams after burying my husband. As a result, my celebration party consisted of Gary, who was four weeks old, and Mam.

In hindsight, I should have questioned a lot of things. You see one of them, you see them all. That was one of the things we said. I perceived Clodagh and Alan as an extremely close and happy couple, two sides of the same coin. They and their boys were a happy, wholesome and perfect family. I envied not having the same with Richie.

And even if I found Alan unbearable, it was clear he was worshipped locally. One rare occasion I was at mass, I recall the priest praised him from the altar, calling him 'Master Hawe'. As deputy principal of a national school in a rural area, he was a big fish in a small pond.

So, I never tackled anything, even Alan's behaviour towards me. I didn't want to rock the boat because I knew they would close ranks. And I wanted to see the boys. I loved them and I wanted Gary to grow up knowing them. And if that meant buttoning my lip, that was what I had to do.

I knew I couldn't win a row with them. I believed they held me at arm's length because they didn't approve of me or my lifestyle. I enjoyed a drink and went to pubs. Sometimes I went clubbing. They did none of those things and made me feel like a reprobate for being normal. So I always tried to seek their approval rather than challenge anything. I never saw the red flags or, at least, I didn't recognise them. The truth is, I'd never heard of 'coercive control'. I had no clue what it meant.

Clodagh and I had a few moments before she died when it looked like we were growing closer again. I didn't know it then, but she was becoming disillusioned with Alan Hawe and beginning to realise he was not everything she had thought him to be.

Gerry's sixtieth birthday took place in June. Clodagh collected me, and the two of us turned out to be wearing dresses in the same colour. She looked elegant in a peach dress with a shawl over it, pinned with a cameo brooch. I wore a short peach dress that was fit for Club V, the nightclub in Virginia at the time. I burst out laughing as I compared the two of us. 'Clodagh, we look like we're going to two very different events!' She laughed, too, and told me I looked stunning.

It was a lovely summer evening, and Gerry had erected a giant inflatable pub in the back garden. Mam had been sick, and she barely made it out of hospital in time for the party. That night, Clodagh and I watched through the Perspex window of the blow-up bar as Mam gave it socks on the dance floor. We wrapped our arms around each other and laughed. 'Isn't she some woman?' Clodagh said. It was a little moment between us and one of the few we'd had since Alan Hawe arrived in our lives.

That evening, we were all inside the 'bouncy boozer' as Gerry cut the cake. There was a lot of hilarity, drinking, cheering and jeering going on. The night was brilliant fun. And there, in the background, behind Gerry and Carmel and all the cake-cutting antics, I happened to notice Alan Hawe. He was in one of the seats at the back of the bar, disengaged from everyone and everything around him. He was expressionless, just sitting there, observing everyone.

That was the way he was. He was quieter than most people and socially inept. He was a silent presence … but I never perceived him as a physical threat. It was just that I never wanted to be around him. I had no real relationship with him and felt uncomfortable in his company. Years later, I discovered Alan Hawe was even more uneasy around me and regarded me as 'a threat'.

When I rang the house that day in August, ten days before the murders, Clodagh answered and said she was on her own with the boys. I silently thanked the stars that he wasn't there and drove straight over. When we arrived at the house, Gary dashed in to join Niall and Ryan in the playroom. He loved every chance to be with his cousins. I put my head in the door to say hello, and they were already making a big fuss of him. They were such great kids who always included him in whatever they did. He was only three when they died, but he still remembers and talks about them.

I was glad to have some private time with Clodagh. We hadn't shared our feelings in ages. I was always conscious of what she had said: 'If you tell me, you tell Alan.' But it was coming up to Tadhg's anniversary, and his death was weighing on me heavily. I needed to talk to someone who remembered and loved him as I did.

'I can't believe it's almost six years since he's gone,' I said. 'I usually smile when I think about him, but in the last few weeks, I don't know what it is, Clodagh, but I just can't stop crying about him now.'

She understood exactly what I was talking about.

'It comes in waves, Jacqueline,' she said. 'In between, life goes on, and then another wave crashes when you least expect it. It happens to me, too, like that.'

And that afternoon, she said something that has stayed with me ever since. 'Don't ever be defined by what's happened to you, Jacqueline,' she said. 'We shouldn't be defined by what happens to us.'

I remember it so well because I thought it was a strange thing for her to say to me. I wondered afterwards why she had said it. *Clodagh might feel defined by the tragedies in our family, but I don't*, I thought. *I'm doing well. I'm happy rearing Gary and living in my own house. I'm back working with a good job and career. I've moved on. I'm not defined by what happened.*

I didn't think anything of it until Alan Hawe did what he did. Now I think of the last time I saw Clodagh alive and remember her words to me.

11

Sleepwalking

I forgot Niall's glasses. I couldn't believe I left that house of horror without his spectacles. Poor Niall never went anywhere without them. Even though logic told me he would never need glasses again, I couldn't bear to let him go to his eternal rest without them. That was why I had to return to Clodagh's house on Thursday, 1 September, the day before the wake.

I couldn't summon the courage to enter Liam and Niall's room a second time after what I had witnessed. A guard offered to go to his room instead and found the glasses for me. I also found Clodagh's favourite mug while I was waiting in the kitchen. I sped away from the house and drove straight to the funeral home.

I handed Niall's glasses to the funeral director, Declan Finnegan, and kept the mug to bring home to Mam. I thought about Clodagh and the boys lying on the other side of the door. It felt wrong to leave them alone in that room. I also hadn't seen my sister the week before she died and felt regretful for leaving it so long. Now it was too late. I left, feeling guilty and remorseful.

Mam and I got to the funeral home well in advance of the wake, which was due to start at 3 p.m. Mam had decided that she wanted to remember her daughter and grandsons the way she knew them. She couldn't bear to see them laid out.

I made a different decision. Probably in an effort to alleviate my guilt, I decided to walk through those doors to say goodbye to them. Seeing Clodagh, Liam, Niall, Ryan and Alan Hawe in a long succession of coffins was too much. All the light, love and joy that had defined Clodagh and her boys was gone, brutally extinguished. The sight of them all lying there brought home the reality of their loss to me.

I couldn't bear to talk to them or touch them as I'd intended. The only words I spoke were addressed to Alan Hawe: 'What the fuck were you thinking?' I fled the room in tears.

The sense of bleak, endless silence I experienced that morning has stayed with me. For some, seeing the bodies of loved ones helps the grieving process, but I have always profoundly regretted going into that room. I still have flashbacks of how they looked that day.

The day took another turn for the worse when I spotted

my father. Clodagh hadn't spoken to him in years. She'd wanted nothing to do with him, so he had never met Alan or any of his grandchildren. And yet he appeared at the funeral home dressed in a full morning suit. It was the last thing Clodagh would have wanted, so I was horrified. I glanced at Mam, relieved she hadn't seen him. *She's upset enough without him here*, I thought.

I went over to him quietly. 'Look, we don't want you here, and we don't want a scene, so I'm asking you to go.'

But he turned to Declan beside me.

'And who's she?' he said, nodding in my direction.

Well, that says it all, I remember thinking, turning on my heel. My own father didn't recognise me. But I already hurt so badly that I couldn't feel any more pain. I realised he wouldn't go, and I could do nothing about it.

I was more upset about how Clodagh would have felt. The last interaction between Clodagh and our father had taken place outside Cavan courthouse in February 2011 after the inquest into Tadhg's death. I won't go into what led to the showdown, but the colloquial phrase she 'ripped him a new one' is the best description of the event.

Clodagh had a lot to get off her chest and, by God, she did it that day. I stood back in awe of her ferocity. She showed a strength she often concealed. Part of me thought, *We're not that different, really.*

'Jesus, Clodagh, I didn't know you had that in you!' I said to her afterwards.

'You're not the only one who can fight,' she said. Both she and Alan Hawe regarded me as someone who spoke her mind and never held back my opinions. It was one of the moments I was proudest of Clodagh, and we held each other's hand the whole journey home. I still feel bad that I didn't do the same for her on the day of her wake.

Within the hour, another unexpected confrontation arose. As I've said, Mam had made clear she wanted to remember her daughter and grandsons as she'd known them. After my experience hours earlier, I wholeheartedly agreed. We arranged with Declan that the caskets would be closed when the funeral home opened to the public.

Our relationship with the Hawes, such as it was, began to unravel as a result. They arrived just before the funeral home opened to the public and went into the viewing room. Declan came out and spoke quietly to me. 'Jacqueline, the Hawes want to leave the coffins open for the wake.'

'No way, Declan. That won't be happening. Mam doesn't want to see them like that. I don't think it's appropriate to leave the coffins open either.'

I knew some of the boys' young and innocent friends would come to pay their respects. They were too young to be exposed to so much death. I also knew Clodagh would not want the boys or her on public display.

Declan appeared a bit later, his face flushed and brow furrowed. 'Listen, Jacqueline. They're insisting that the coffins be left open.'

I felt my blood pressure rise, and panic set in.

'No, Declan. This is final. While the coffins are open, the Hawes can spend as long as they like with everyone. But the coffins are to be closed before we go in.'

Just as the funeral home was about to open to the public, Declan came to me a third time. 'Please come into the room, Jacqueline, and speak with them yourself. I can't close the coffins.'

I swore under my breath and entered that room again – the last thing I wanted to do. I explained that the coffins must be closed. Mam did not want to see her family like that. And so it was.

The disagreement over the coffin lids caused the first fracture in our relationship with the Hawes.

But I never regretted insisting upon closed coffins. I thought of Clodagh's friends and colleagues coming to pay their respects and the boys' young friends attending. It would have been unnecessarily traumatising to see all the children laid out. Clodagh was incredibly private, with no Facebook, Instagram, Twitter or Snapchat. She never allowed anyone to post photos of her boys on social media. Open coffins were not what she would have wanted.

I went through my phone, searching for photos from happier times of each family member. Declan printed them off and displayed them in frames on the coffins instead. Mam and I sat through the wake, barely able to make eye contact with anyone, wishing it would end. We sat behind a red rope set up by Declan, separating us from people paying their respects. We weren't interacting with anyone, and I don't remember much about who was or wasn't there. I don't remember seeing my father again. I know thousands of people came through the funeral home that evening to pay their respects.

We asked mourners to donate to the country's biggest suicide prevention charity, Pieta House, in place of flowers. That alone shows how skewed our thinking was. Why didn't we ask for donations to Women's Aid or Offaly Domestic Violence Support Service, or another charity supporting victims of violence? As a family, we had only experienced the trauma of suicide, and it was the first charity at the forefront of our minds. We still didn't comprehend what had happened in Clodagh's house.

When I think back now, it seems odd that Mam or I never rethought the funeral arrangements. The fact that Alan Hawe had murdered Clodagh and the boys should have been enough to make us stop and consider what we were doing. But it didn't. Seeing the boys' blood spattered across their bedroom should have made me shout, 'No!' But even that didn't do it.

It didn't help that most of the information about the murders was still being withheld from us. We hadn't read Alan Hawe's murder letter. I still didn't know anything about the man he really was. Alan had painted a picture of himself as a devoted father and husband. It was difficult for us to see beyond that carefully crafted image. We still thought of him as a great father and husband, a man Clodagh loved and trusted.

He was also above reproach in the community. He was the respectable vice-principal of a school, a treasurer in the local GAA, a mass-going communicant, a reader at mass and a great friend of the local priest. He didn't drink, smoke or gamble, and had nothing to do with drugs. Along with Clodagh, he was a good provider for his family, and his wife and children thought the world of him.

My mother's revelation that he was viewing porn came as a shock because it was boring, staid and sensible Alan. We were still a long way from discovering the truth, but Alan did not fit the bill of a leering porn addict. Nor could we see him as a cruel, savage man who would axe and knife his wife and children to death. The picture I still had in my head was of Alan, the tortured man, who had accumulated so much pain, possibly at work, that he snapped under the pressure. He had exploded like a pressure cooker, destroying all around him.

We avoided all the coverage of the murders. Mam and our immediate family looked away, and maybe that was a mistake. We weren't even aware yet that Alan Hawe was centre stage in the news, being eulogised by some as a near saint. I've since seen Father Kelly's quotes that 'Master Hawe' of Castlerahan national school was highly regarded in the community. Locals described him to the media as 'the most normal person you could meet' and 'the best teacher in the world'. Everyone piled on praise for Alan Hawe in the days after the murders, and I understand that. They only knew the person he presented to them, just as Mam and I did.

I've since seen some of the newspaper headlines from that time. According to one, 'They lost a true gentleman', while *The Irish Times* read, 'Wonderful children who will be greatly missed.' The *Irish Independent* asked, 'How could he kill those boys?' We had no idea that week that Clodagh was missing from the narrative.

We were also unaware that people such as Gary Gannon, then a Social Democrats councillor in Dublin, were asking, 'What about their mother?' He wrote an article titled 'Her Name Is Clodagh' on the morning of her wake. He and others began to complain that Clodagh had disappeared in the avalanche of media coverage. If someone had said #HerNameIsClodagh had gone viral on social media, I might have woken up. But we didn't hear anything about it until the following week, maybe even two weeks after the funeral.

For us, nothing was adding up, nothing was making sense, and nobody was telling us anything. I was in a stupor. Mam was too. And not a single person said to me, 'Is this wise? Burying a murderer with his victims?' We might have rethought the funeral arrangements if anyone suggested that he shouldn't be buried with them. If we'd had another few days, if we hadn't bowed to pressure from Father Kelly to have the funeral so quickly, the reality that Alan Hawe murdered my sister and nephews might have percolated through. Savagely murdered them.

Even looking at Alan Hawe in the funeral home and seeing what he'd done to my sister and my three little nephews, I still didn't think, *Don't bury him with them*. I was in a state of suspended disbelief, I know now. All that ran through my mind was, *Is this really happening?*

But it doesn't stop the guilt that remains to this day. All I can do is put it down to shock and trauma and what they do to your brain. Rational decision-making was difficult, and my reasoning faculties seemed to freeze. Somehow, I continued to sleepwalk into one of the worst mistakes I had ever made in my life.

12

Funeral

The sky was low and steely grey as the cortège left the funeral home for Castlerahan church on Saturday, 3 September. We drove slowly through Cavan town, a sombre procession of five hearses, three bearing white coffins, and I remember the streets lined with people, most of whom we didn't know. Hundreds, maybe thousands, came out in a show of respect for Clodagh and the boys.

The long line of hearses left Cavan and continued snaking along the country roads until we reached Ballyjamesduff, and it was the same there. The whole of Ballyjamesduff town closed that day, and it was staggering to see so many people lining the streets. The vast crowds along the route all the way to Castlerahan seemed incredible, almost as unimaginable as burying my sister and my three little nephews. Everything felt surreal, and it was impossible to accept what was happening. *I'm about to bury Liam. I'm about to bury Clodagh and the boys.*

I sat in the front seat of the hearse that carried Liam, and Liam's driver followed the lead funeral car containing Mam with Clodagh's remains. Behind Liam was Niall's hearse and Ryan's, with Alan Hawe's at the rear. Crowds of people came into view as we approached Castlerahan church from the Ballyjamesduff Road. So many mourners descended that locals had turned the fields surrounding the church into makeshift car parks. Sometimes the media shows footage of the hearses coming down that hill, and I have to glance away. The pain it brings back is overwhelming.

The hearse carrying Clodagh swung slowly left through the church gates, and the sea of people parted to let the car ascend the hill to the doors of St Mary's.

Liam's driver waited outside the gates until the lead hearse cleared the hill and then went to follow, but the car stalled. He turned the key in the ignition. Nothing.

'Jesus, there's not a gig out of it,' he said. He panicked. People passing stared through the windows, and I gazed ahead, my vision blurred with tears.

'It'll be okay. Just give it a second and try again.'

The tears ran unchecked down my face as the driver tried the ignition again and again. All I could think was, *Liam doesn't want to go. This is poor Liam's way of saying he doesn't want to go.* I was trying to connect to those I'd lost. The funeral was another ordeal in this horrendous, endless nightmare, and I wanted to scream at the injustice of it all. *Jesus Christ, Liam, this shouldn't be happening to any of you. I'm so sorry we let this happen.* More guilt.

The other hearses started passing our stalled one, and the driver got out, seeking help to carry Liam's coffin to the church. My eyes were burning as I followed. I heard the burst of a camera shutter before I saw a photographer somehow hanging from a telegraph pole. I felt so exposed. Even writing this, my heart beats faster thinking about that camera and the incessant clicking.

But the sight of the church looming above made it all too real for me. I thought of Liam behind me and didn't think I would reach the church door. My head felt light, and my legs started to sway. I thought I was about to faint when, out of nowhere, my cousin Melissa reached out for me. A kind garda propped me on my other side. They helped me up the hill to the church door where Mam was already alarmed, wondering where I was.

As we entered the dimly lit St Mary's, we saw the Hawes and their relatives filling the seats on one side of the aisle. We poured into the pews on the other side. The coffins stretched across the altar – three white ones in the middle, two adult-sized oak ones on either side. The little church was packed to capacity, and hundreds more congregated outside as they relayed the funeral ceremony over loudspeakers. The doors were jammed with people, so no fresh air made its way inside.

The now-retired bishop of Kilmore, Dr Leo O'Reilly, flanked Father Kelly, who recalled visits to Clodagh's house during his homily. 'Clodagh with her scones, red jam and mug of coffee. Liam, Niall and Ryan busy like budding engineers, building all kinds of Lego. Alan standing with his back to the kitchen sink, totally at ease enjoying the *bean an tí* and the antics of unspoilt and respectful sons ...'

The church had been an integral part of their lives. Clodagh and Alan did the readings on Sundays; Liam and Niall were altar servers, and all three boys were choir singers. They had watched as Richie and I made our vows at the same altar. They were also there for Richie's funeral and Gary's christening. The previous Sunday morning, just hours before Alan Hawe had murdered them, they sat together in their usual pew near the front of the church. And now they were lined up in coffins on the same altar.

'There is a dark side too,' said Father Kelly. 'How could so much goodness be destroyed? How could so much happiness be invaded? It is not for us to seek answers or to surmise about behaviour. We are all trying to cope with a tragedy beyond our understanding ...'

Even in my stupor of grief and bewilderment, I remember hearing his words, 'It is not for us to seek answers,' and thought, *Why wouldn't we want answers? Of course, we want answers.*

Mam placed a family portrait on Clodagh's coffin as an offertory gift. A basketball was placed on Liam's coffin, and Niall's sports trophy stood on his. Granddad Gerry, as he was known to Ryan, placed a fluffy dog on the smallest white coffin to represent Ryan's affection and innocence. Someone from Alan Hawe's side brought up a Kilkenny jersey for his coffin.

After communion, I read the poem 'The Broken Chain' by Ron Tranmer. The words in the final verse resonated with me about how the chain will link again in heaven.

'Sleep tight,' I managed to utter, through the ball of grief lodged in my throat. I remember the smell of incense as Father Kelly swung the thurible around all the coffins. My body was racked by one crying jag after another. I couldn't trust myself with Ryan's coffin, and I abandoned plans to help carry him the few metres around the side of the church to his grave. I'm glad I didn't try. Seeing the vast expanse of green canvas covering the five burial plots was like another blow to the pit of my stomach.

Nothing prepared me either for the scene of the grave-diggers lowering the coffins, one by one, into the ground. As each one went down, it was like a stab to the heart. I thought I must be numb to pain for ever after, and tears blinded me again as five white doves were released. We watched them fluttering before rising, circling in the sky above us and flying away. It was one upsetting horror after another. Most of the time, I stood swaying at the gravesides on that gloomy autumnal evening, wondering, *What the fuck is happening?*

And then it was all over, and people were milling around again. A frenzy of activity and pressing crowds surrounded us, and Mam fled. She was too upset, unable to bear any more heartfelt condolences or sympathies. There were so many people that I lost her in the crowd.

I'd seen media before at funerals, but never anything like the crowd that day. Cameras and journalists surrounded the church, making it seem a circus instead of a funeral. I felt our family was like a zoo exhibit or some bit-player in a tragic soap in which we'd never wanted a part. For the first time, I wished I had listened to Mam when she suggested that we have a private family funeral. I wasn't even sure what a private funeral would look like, but I argued that it wouldn't be fair to Clodagh's or the boys' friends, especially Liam's from Virginia community school. They needed an opportunity to grieve. But I realised I had made a mistake. A private funeral would have been the right thing to do.

For a few minutes, I panicked when I couldn't find the rest of the family, Mam, Carmel, Gerry and my cousins, Melissa, Audrey and Eileen. We eventually met at the bottom of the road. We returned to Carmel and Gerry's house, where many of our other close relatives and friends gathered. Mam was on the phone, trying to call the Hawes to invite them to join us. She had given them her house that weekend while she stayed with me. She couldn't reach them, and we heard later they were in the community hall up the road from the church. My father was there too.

The next day, Alan Hawe's brothers came to the house to return Mam's keys to us. Stephen Hawe had already returned to Kilkenny, but his wife sat in the car. I went out to say goodbye to her.

And then they left, and the long silence we had experienced before the funeral resumed. We waited until the afternoon when the Sunday masses were over before returning to the cemetery. We were relieved to find it deserted and the churchyard empty of cars. The only sound was the familiar rustling of leaves and the soft coos of pigeons. We stood there silently for ages, gazing at the carpet of white roses wilting on the five raised mounds of soil. I remember glancing at Mam and thinking how ill she looked, so pale and drawn. Her skin was nearly translucent. And as I looked at the expanse of graves in front of us, realisation hit me like a sledgehammer.

In the calm and silence of the graveyard, my reasoning finally returned. I thought of Clodagh in the ground with Liam, Niall and Ryan, and I thought of Alan Hawe in there with them, and my stomach lurched.

What have we done? I thought. *Jesus Christ, what have we done?* My head was spinning, but Mam was in enough turmoil, so I didn't dare give voice to the horror I felt.

Clodagh must have spoken to both of us at that moment because Mam lifted her eyes from the devastating scene around us. She looked at me in shock and uttered the exact words running through my head. 'What have we done?' she said.

13

Exhumation

Mam and I clutched each other's hands and buried them in the sofa cushion between us. Gerry and Carmel sat on the other couch, and Stephen and Olive Hawe took seats that faced us. My heart beat so loudly I thought the whole room could hear it. I was afraid I might vomit. How do you tell a mother and father that you want their son removed from your family's grave?

Two weeks after the funeral, we met with the Hawes to broach the subject of having Alan Hawe exhumed from the grave in Castlerahan. They were coming anyway to make statements to gardaí in Bailieborough, and we asked them to call to us on the way.

Understandably, perhaps, the meeting didn't go well. The Hawes were shocked and argued that our move was precipitous because the investigation wasn't over. As it continued, tempers frayed. The Hawes pointed out that they had had nothing to do with the funeral arrangements, that we had watched Alan Hawe being buried, and that was that. It was too late now. What were they to do with him? And one word borrowed another. Temperatures and voices rose.

Carmel sat poised and dignified as the lady she is, but I saw Gerry, his colour high, running a hand around the back of his neck. He had heard enough. He turned to Stephen Hawe and said, 'I don't care what you do with him. Put him in a freezer, but he's coming out of there!' Gerry and Carmel always have our backs.

Gerry always said what needed saying with no frills. But that was the first time in my life that I'd ever seen such anger in him. That comment did not come from malice. His anger was born of protectiveness for Mam and me and his love for us, Clodagh and the boys. He has always been the male role model in our family, and he loved the boys so much.

At that stage, the Hawes left. Where do we go from here? The gardaí said it had nothing to do with them, and solicitors said the same. The county council said exhumation was only possible if the deceased person's next of kin asks for the remains to be moved. The law was on the Hawes' side. The grave was in our name, but they were the only ones who could move Alan Hawe out of it. We weren't sure what we could do to move the issue of exhumation forward.

Soon we had heard enough to know that the murders were not an impulsive, pressure-cooker explosion in which Alan Hawe had gone temporarily mad. With a sense of growing horror, we started to understand that this was a meticulously planned evil deed.

We still didn't have access to Alan Hawe's murder letter, but what we gleaned from our family liaison officer and the media helped us realise how extensive his 'note' was. We thought of the jewellery laid out on the bed and Clodagh's dressy shoes on the bedroom floor.

We thought of how he had murdered Clodagh, creeping up behind her with an axe, and realised that that was only possible because he had rearranged the furniture just before the murders.

Throughout all the years they had lived in that house, the room never changed. You walked through the kitchen's glass double doors to enter the living room. Clodagh had turned it into a beautiful, cosy room. She had framed the panoramic window overlooking the countryside with long cream curtains. Underneath the window was her terracotta bouclé couch, decorated with cream embroidered cushions and warm wool throws. She had a ceramic lamp on a side table beside the couch, which glowed with warmth in the evening. Anyone sitting on the couch could see everyone enter or approach from the kitchen.

But two weeks earlier Alan Hawe had rearranged everything so that the back of the couch faced the double doors from the kitchen. Clodagh explained the suite had to be moved because Alan wanted to bring in the piano from the playroom. He said the temperature there wasn't right for it. But it meant that on the night of the murders, as Clodagh sat on the couch, she was unaware of Hawe approaching from behind with an axe.

In twelve years, nothing had changed in that house, and two weeks before he murdered them all, he rearranged the furniture.

We asked so many questions we began turning into detectives. We tried to fathom how he had got hold of the axe, which was normally stored in the shed. He must have brought it in and hidden it in the kitchen beforehand. Clodagh would have asked where he was going if he'd gone out to get it that night. I had a reading with a medium who told me about a weapon under the bed. I never mentioned wondering about the axe, but maybe that was where he stashed it. All I know is that it must have been in the house beforehand.

We began to realise Alan Hawe had methodically set about annihilating his whole family. He might have planned it from the start of the holidays, but he certainly planned for some time to do it before he was due to return to school. Murder was foremost on his mind when he thanked my mother and headed off for a final evening with his family.

Father Kelly arrived at my house unannounced one day in the weeks after the funeral. I rang Mam, and she drove to meet us there. Father Kelly had lauded Alan Hawe as a great family man before and during the funeral, and we were determined he wouldn't do it again at the month's mind. But he tried to dismiss our feelings about his continued praise for Alan Hawe.

'The poor man couldn't have been in his right mind. Sure, wasn't he a great father and husband all those years?'

'He was, Father, right up until the moment he murdered them all,' I said.

But Father Kelly seemed to think Alan Hawe had done nothing wrong. Or if he had, that it wasn't his fault.

We shouldn't have been surprised. Clodagh had said the priest would often walk past her in the house as if she was invisible. She was 'the little woman', and he was only interested in talking to 'Master Hawe'.

'Alan Hawe is a murderer,' I said finally. 'We want you to say that what he did was evil, and if you don't, we'll walk out of that church.'

Father Kelly visibly bristled, and his eyes narrowed. 'I will not be bullied into blackening Alan's name,' he said icily.

He clearly didn't accept that Alan's name was blackened the moment he knifed his innocent wife and children.

'Well, then, Father, you're going to have a battle on your hands,' I said. 'Whatever happened to the commandment, You shall not kill?'

We didn't have to storm out of the church during the month's mind after all. Father Kelly must have decided he didn't want a scene, so the word 'evil' duly appeared in connection with Alan Hawe in his sermon. However, he made clear that he didn't want Alan Hawe moved from the grave either. 'I don't agree with you exhuming Alan,' he said, when he heard our plans. 'But I won't stand in your way.'

He couldn't have stood in our way if he'd wanted to.

Nearly a month after the month's mind, on 13 October, we marked Ryan's seventh birthday. Mam thought the Hawes might have cooled down and be open to discussing the exhumation again. She tried to make contact and was told that it was best if future contact was made through their solicitor.

Our next time seeing the Hawes was November when the guards called us to another meeting to update us. Stephen and Olive Hawe, Mam and I and a couple of other guards, including our family liaison officer, gathered in a room in Bailieborough garda station, an old shale stone building on Barrack Street. The atmosphere between the two families was understandably frosty.

We learnt Alan Hawe had been looking at more than images of naked women from the waist up. The guards told us he had been looking at many pornographic websites. They also said they believed the pornography was an issue between him and Clodagh. We started asking about the nature of the pornography, but one garda was very dismissive.

'It's not porn as we know it,' he said. The impression we got was of something incidental or minor. But, as we were to discover later, it wasn't pornography as most people know it. It was far worse.

The guards told us they had examined Clodagh's computer and that she had been researching 'parenting alone at Christmas' in December 2015. She had also been researching teaching jobs abroad in Dubai in March 2016. This wasn't entirely accurate as we were to learn later. But for the first time, I realised that Clodagh was actively considering leaving Alan Hawe. She had been exploring the possibility of a life apart from him in the year before she was murdered. At that stage, I turned and appealed to the Hawes to allow us to exhume the body.

But they did not wish to reconsider until the investigation was complete.

The guards moved on. They informed us that a post-mortem carried out by Deputy State Pathologist Dr Michael Curtis found that Hawe's thyroid gland revealed traces of a rare disease, Hashimoto's thyroiditis. He said there could be a connection between this disease 'in the acute phase' and 'psychiatric illness including psychosis'.

However, the post-mortem had shown no evidence of Alan Hawe being in an 'acute phase' of any neurological disease. Also, much of the evidence, including the organised nature of the killings, contradicted any notion that Hawe had psychosis. If this was an acute episode, how could he have carried it out in such a meticulous and controlled fashion?

I called the coroner to ask about Hashimoto's thyroiditis in the days after our meeting, and she dismissed the findings as 'a red herring'. Despite this, the post-mortem report prompted her to seek a new report on Alan Hawe, which delayed the inquest process for months. The issue of Hashimoto's thyroiditis was irrelevant, but it muddied the waters for a while.

I also remember asking the guards to see Alan Hawe's murder letter again in Bailieborough that day and being told, 'No, it's evidence.' In hindsight, I'd ask, 'Evidence for what?' There was no trial and there was never going to be one as the perpetrator was dead.

Unexpectedly, a few days later, our solicitor said that the Hawes agreed in principle to exhume their son. Furthermore, they were starting the application process to have him moved. I exhaled with relief.

We started to hear more information about the night of the murders. The levels of coldness and depravity still defy description. Alan Hawe was a wolf in sheep's clothing who fooled us all.

Hours after killing his wife and sons, Hawe transferred money from a joint bank account with Clodagh to an account in his name only. It was further confirmation that these were calculated and planned murders. How else could a man who had stabbed his wife and children sit down at his computer afterwards, recall all his passwords and calmly transfer funds?

We also learnt that succession law allowed the perpetrator of a spousal homicide to be the beneficiary of the couple's assets. As he was the surviving spouse, he inherited everything, including the family home. After his suicide, his family were the sole beneficiaries of his and Clodagh's estate.

As we heard more and more damning information about Alan Hawe, we became increasingly disturbed by his presence in the grave with Clodagh and the boys.

Yet the months dragged on, and there was no sign of the exhumation. The Hawe family's solicitor insisted no one was dragging their heels. He explained the family had to apply for an exhumation licence to Cavan County Council. They also had to involve Environmental Health in a ground inspection, then receive an exhumation order from the coroner. All these had to be delivered to the funeral director in Kilkenny before the exhumation could begin.

In March, seven months after the murders, we asked that the body be removed ahead of Clodagh's fortieth birthday on Easter Sunday, 16 April. At the end of March our hearts sank when we were told the ground inspection hadn't been passed. So, Clodagh's fortieth birthday came and went, May arrived, and Alan Hawe was still in the grave with her.

It came to the stage where I could not bear to look at that name on that cross. Its presence goaded me. Out of sheer frustration, I managed to yank it out of the ground and throw it into a six-foot-deep drain behind the graves.

It made me feel better for a while. The parish priest went ballistic, trying to find out who had done it, and he got Declan Finnegan to put the cross back.

Declan rang me, asking, 'Do you know anything about this, Jacqueline?' I'm sure he didn't want the job of fishing that cross out of a drain and putting it back in place.

'No,' I said. 'I've no idea what you're talking about.'

Yanking out the grave marker was not my finest moment but it was my way of coping at the time. Hawe's continued presence there with Clodagh and the boys made me depressed. I blamed myself for him being there in the first place. I hated myself for allowing it to happen. But the decision to move him was totally in the Hawe family's hands. We were powerless.

In desperation, I rang Environmental Health in Cavan one day to beg them to allow the exhumation. After I'd convinced them I was Clodagh's sister, they confirmed that the ground inspection had passed in March, three weeks before Clodagh's birthday. Stunned, I rang the coroner, and she said the exhumation order had been issued on the same day. I don't know why there was such a delay, but I rang the Hawes in a fury. I made my feelings very plain.

Within days, we got news from gardaí that the exhumation was happening on Wednesday, 10 May 2017. I felt like slumping to the ground with relief. But the lead detective in the investigation said a court order prevented me attending the event. I should have demanded to see that court order, but when I objected, he said he would allow me to be at the exhumation if the family liaison officer also attended. I shrugged. I was happy to agree to that condition. We were told the exhumation would start at 8 a.m. and take ten hours to complete.

'Ten hours?' I said to Mam. 'Sure, how could it take that long?'

The family liaison officer arranged to collect me from my house at 7.30 a.m. that Wednesday. However, at six thirty that morning, Gerry called me from the graveyard. 'You'd better get out here quick,' he said. 'He's on his way out.'

The blood drained from me, but now I think back and laugh at his blunt words.

He explained later that he and Carmel had gone to the graveyard early because he suspected something was afoot. Castlerahan national school was across the road from the church and the cemetery.

'They'd hardly open the grave in front of a school full of kids on a Wednesday morning,' he said. He was right. When he arrived, the gravediggers and gardaí had been on site for almost an hour.

Gary was staying with my cousin overnight, so I could leave my house and drive from Virginia to Castlerahan on two wheels without any family liaison officer. It was clear they had never meant for us to be at the exhumation. By then, I had contact numbers for a few media people. I rang them and tipped off everyone I could.

When I arrived, privacy screens had been erected, concealing all the activity at the grave. Officials from Environmental Health and Cavan County Council were standing around. Gardaí were also there, with the funeral director and his men, maybe six or seven people in all.

None of the guards mentioned a court order or asked me for the family liaison officer. Instead, they shook my hand. Carmel, Gerry and I stood a short distance away, and Seamus Enright, from the local paper *Anglo-Celt*, joined us soon after. Someone from a national paper also arrived in time.

I remember it being a bright morning, yet I felt very cold. I don't know whether it was the early-morning chill or because of all the anxiety I was experiencing. For my own sanity, I needed to see Alan Hawe being removed to believe it really happened. Within half an hour or so of my arrival, the body was exhumed. I would have missed everything if I'd gone at the appointed hour.

We watched silently as Alan Hawe was loaded into a waiting silver Toyota HiAce van. 'Gerrup there, ya hoor ya!' one guard muttered as Hawe's remains were heaved into the van. I would have smiled, but I was crying tears of relief that, after more than eight months of fighting, Hawe had been removed from our family grave. Of course, that relief was only short-lived because his absence changed nothing. Clodagh and her boys were still dead, but at least they could rest in peace without him beside them: we had undone the bad decisions we'd made. It didn't salve my conscience or relieve the guilt I felt for putting him there in the first place, but it was one less battle to fight. Little did I think that we'd have another seven-year struggle ahead of us to uncover the truth of what had happened on 29 August.

The Hawes' solicitor released a statement saying, 'The timing of the exhumation was decided by the professionals who dealt with the exhumation' and 'There was no substance to any suggestion that it was delayed for any reason by the Hawes.'

We heard that the family planned to cremate Alan Hawe as he had requested in his murder letter, and they were bringing him to Glasnevin cemetery in Dublin for that purpose. That's as much as we know. And, to be honest, we don't care. To make doubly sure he was gone for ever, we concreted over the grave shortly after he was exhumed. We only cared that he was gone.

14

Confessional Privilege

The parochial house is a few hundred metres up the hill from Castlerahan church. An old country house, it's rendered and painted white with black trim and sheltered by a stone wall and a circle of ancient, towering trees. As I knocked on the door in March 2017, my heart thumped with anxiety.

Alan Hawe's murder letter had prompted the lead detective to declare that whatever had occurred at the school was the catalyst for the murders. Yet Father Kelly, the chairperson of the board of management for the school and a close friend of Alan Hawe, declined to make a statement to the gardaí. So, too, did some board members of Castlerahan national school.

The guards constantly reminded me that their inquiry was not a criminal investigation. Once the perpetrator is dead, there is no trial. Instead, the team relied on witnesses to give voluntary statements. However, the parish priest was the last person I expected to refuse to cooperate with an investigation into the murders of a mother and three children.

'Father Kelly has his own reasons,' the guards said. 'We did try appealing to his conscience, but he pleaded confessional privilege.'

To me, confessional privilege was restricted to anything confided during the sacrament of penance. According to Alan Hawe, he was involved in a series of incidents in the school that year that had little to do with the confession box.

I would later come to understand that what he was reporting to my sister was not the full truth. Yes, there were incidents in the school, which the second investigation would come to uncover, but what Hawe was disclosing to Clodagh placed himself erroneously in the role of victim – he was trying to manipulate her sympathies.

In June 2016, just before the school closed for the summer, I called to see Clodagh. We sat down for coffee, but she was fidgety, getting up and down from her chair, glancing out the window and pacing the kitchen. I could see she was distracted. Clodagh was very private, especially about anything to do with her husband, but something was bothering her. I asked her straight out what was wrong.

She was hesitant at first, and then it all poured out. 'Alan's up with Father Kelly. There's stuff going on in the school.'

'What stuff?'

Clodagh said one of his colleagues had accused him of bullying.

'Alan?' That seemed unlikely to me. Hawe was acting principal when I was studying for my post-grad after Richie died. During that time, he had asked me to devise a bullying and harassment policy for the school.

Clodagh said it had started over a new school rule that stated any child who wet the toilet floor had to clean up their mess. According to Alan Hawe's version of events, Little Ryan had gone in and seen that the floor was wet. He'd come out and told the teacher, and the teacher made him go in and clean it. It escalated from there. Hawe said he tried to address this but was told if he wanted to talk to a teacher about his child, he'd have to make an appointment like every other parent.

When he went to speak to the principal, some disagreement broke out. Hawe claimed the principal accused him of bullying her and barricading her in the room. He told Clodagh that the principal then left the school, and he presumed she had gone straight to Father Kelly's house because she didn't return for hours.

'That's all a bit dramatic over a wet toilet floor, isn't it?' I remember saying to Clodagh.

Clodagh never found out what happened. When she said she wanted to meet with the school to discuss what had happened, Alan refused to let her near the place. It all seemed like a storm in a teacup, but Clodagh believed him and was very worried. When Alan Hawe arrived back from visiting Father Kelly. The first thing Clodagh said to him, and I remember it distinctly, was 'I'm sorry, Alan. I've had to tell Jacqueline.'

Hawe nodded but didn't volunteer anything about his meeting with Father Kelly. I felt sympathy for them because they were clearly distressed about events.

'Alan, I'm really sorry,' I said. 'From what I've heard, this sounds crazy.' God, I even put my arm around him. Every time I think about that now, I want to chop it off. I feel foolish for not having seen through him – I would later come to realise how events got blown out of all proportion in the darkness of Hawe's mind.

'We'll sort this out,' I assured him.

I left shortly after, and the incident was never spoken about again. I assumed it was sorted because the summer holidays started, and Clodagh didn't mention it after that. I knew he didn't like her telling me anything, so I never intruded in Clodagh's business. It was the only time I tried to bond with Hawe.

Now, here we were, six months since Clodagh and the boys were murdered, and we still didn't know what, if anything, his colleague or Hawe had told Father Kelly. We needed to know what had happened at the school. Why did Hawe repeatedly refer to the school in his murder letter? Why did he kill my sister and her three boys the night before he was due to return to work? It didn't make sense that the murder spree was over a row about Ryan and a toilet floor.

It grew increasingly apparent, however, that he had spun a web of lies to Clodagh and everyone else he encountered. I needed the school's and Father Kelly's help if Mam and I were ever to uncover what had prompted Alan Hawe to commit that evil act.

So, when I knocked on the door of the parochial house that evening, it was to plead for the parish priest to disclose what information he had.

In his late seventies, Father Kelly was a heavyset, short man with a good head of grey hair and a bulbous nose. He was a man's man who loved the GAA and Gaelic football, and appeared to have little time for or interest in women. After the row Mam and I had had with him over the month's mind, I knew Father Kelly would hold a grudge. He wouldn't be receptive to my plea for information, but I had to try.

First, I talked to him about Richie's fourth-anniversary mass the following month. Then I broached his refusal to make a statement.

'If you won't tell the gardaí, please just tell me what happened,' I said.

Father Kelly's tone was immediately cold and clipped. 'As I've already said to the gardaí, that information is confessional privilege.'

I continued pleading. 'I'm not asking you to break the seal of the confessional,' I said. 'We only need to know what happened in the school. Or what Alan Hawe told you happened. Can't you do that?'

'Anything Alan Hawe told me is private.'

'But it's not confessional privilege.'

'I decide what's confessional privilege, not you,' he said.

My frustration grew. The priest had information we needed, and his refusal to help the investigation hindered everything. The school had released a statement saying Alan Hawe had not been facing a threat of disciplinary action. Yet we knew he had contacted his union, the Irish National Teachers' Organisation.

'Clodagh and the boys are murdered. Alan Hawe is dead. Who are you protecting? What is there to hide at this stage?'

His expression was stone cold. 'No one is going to make me reveal confidential communications between me and anyone in my parish. That is my decision, and I won't be changing my mind.'

So, that was that. I gathered up my things and left with tears in my eyes, baffled by his undying loyalty to a man who had murdered a woman and three children.

Father Felim Kelly remained true to his word. He died in Cavan general hospital on 1 May 2019, and brought to his grave any information or insights he could have provided about Alan Hawe and the murders.

But that was more than two years later. In all that time I could never, for one minute, anticipate what Father Kelly would do.

15

The Counsellor's Notes

I read and reread the words in front of me in disbelief, still unable to absorb the line. The document was typed, so I knew I wasn't misreading the sentence. It was just six simple words, but it was so incompatible with the man's sober façade and his air of conservative respectability that I couldn't take it in.

Alan Hawe tried on Clodagh's underwear.

'On top of everything else, he was a cross-dresser?' I exclaimed.

During a phone call to our then solicitor at the end of April 2017, we discovered she had received summary notes written by Alan Hawe's counsellor. They were among a bundle of documents she had received before the inquest.

We had received little or no information about the murders from the guards via our family liaison officer. We began to see him less as a point of contact and information and more as a buffer between the investigation team and us.

So, of course, we immediately asked the solicitor for a copy of the notes, and she obliged, posting them from her office. Even then, we were nearly expecting them to be intercepted by the guards. They seemed determined to keep us in the dark as much as possible, and for a long time after receiving them, we were afraid to mention that we had these documents.

As soon as the postman dropped the solicitor's envelope through the door, my mother called me. We sat in her house to scour the counsellor's notes and the accompanying garda report. They amounted to four typed A4 pages.

The report revealed the counsellor had refused to hand over his notes after the murders. He cited client confidentiality and produced a contract of confidentiality that he and Alan Hawe had signed. The counsellor's notes were subsequently obtained by the garda investigation.

The notes revealed that Alan Hawe had attended ten sessions with the counsellor in Cavan, on Tuesdays from 15 March until 21 June, just two months before the murders. The counsellor's notes were minimal. The accompanying garda report also says his handwriting was hard to decipher, so they had been typed up for the inquest. Each session amounted to a date and brief jottings – a few words, sometimes a list of terms and short sentences. All the notes were written from the counsellor's memory after each appointment.

The counsellor stated that Alan Hawe came for counselling because of his shame at viewing pornography. Hawe also said he wanted to get his relationship back on track with Clodagh.

For the first session, on 15 March 2016, Alan Hawe arrived with a note containing scribbled travel directions to the counsellor's office. Down the side of these directions were the words 'DVD, Dress, Video, School 12345', and a few people's names. It would be seven years before we understood the meaning behind some of these words and names.

In these notes, the counsellor describes Alan Hawe as 'distressed and full of shame' because he watched porn. Hawe claimed it was all accidental. He had been on internet sites 'getting images for the St Brigid's Cross for school when porn images would come up on the screen'.

'Oh, come on!' I said, upon reading that. 'Who does he think he's fooling?'

The only reason Alan Hawe saw pop-ups was because he was on pornographic sites. He fed lies to his counsellor from the very beginning.

The following week's session concerned aspects of Hawe's relationship with Clodagh. He spoke about Clodagh's upset over discovering he was watching pornography. I didn't need a counsellor's help to understand why Clodagh made Alan Hawe seek help.

Another woman might not have seen Alan Hawe's behaviour as a big problem, but Clodagh and her husband lived in a bubble, a tight-knit family unit. They barely interacted outside that bubble apart from work, his involvement with the GAA and going to mass. For Clodagh, it felt like a betrayal when she discovered her husband was viewing pornography. She asked him to stop, but he continued.

Porn addiction was massive for her because it eroded their physical and emotional intimacy. We all know when something is amiss in a relationship. Her gut told her something was wrong, but she would never be able to help their relationship because she had no clue about the extent of his problems.

He lied to her all the time, manipulating and controlling her to the end.

The words 'sex performance anxiety' appear in the notes for the 5 April session and repeatedly appear in the following sessions. It's known that men addicted to porn find it increasingly difficult to become naturally stimulated. Therapists and medical doctors refer to this side effect of porn addiction as 'porn-induced erectile dysfunction' or PIED. Perhaps if he'd confessed the truth and admitted his addiction to his counsellor or his doctor, they might have been able to help.

Hawe attended his GP about his issues, but she was never aware that he was also seeing a counsellor for his obsession with porn. He kept that hidden from her. He underwent a whole battery of tests with his doctor, and when everything came up clear, she prescribed Viagra.

The notes for that day documented that Hawe claimed a person known to us attempted suicide. I gasped when I read that. The incident never happened, but it allowed him to raise the topic of suicide, and this emerged as a clear pattern in these sessions.

For the 12 April session, the notes are sketchy, but it seemed Hawe talked about the boys' tests and studies as issues of concern. 'Alan has to help Liam study'; 'Liam + test results' and 'Bad piano results'. I had always regarded Alan Hawe as a devoted but over-demanding father. In hindsight, his relentless anxiety about the boys' performance at school and on the sports field were another aspect of his controlling nature. He was overly concerned because he considered their successes or failures a reflection of him.

For 26 April, the notes read: 'Alan said that Clodagh said he should talk about [a relative's] attempted suicide when Alan was 21.' Apparently suicide was all that they discussed on this date and was one of the topics he regularly wanted to revisit.

In his later statement, the counsellor revealed he had explained to Hawe that he had an ethical requirement to break confidentiality if he had reason to believe his patient intended to harm himself or others. He also had a legal requirement to report any disclosures of harm to children. He said that Alan Hawe agreed to work on this basis.

As a result, Hawe would have been careful not to raise any red flags. I wonder whether bringing up the subject of other people's suicides and attempted suicides was his way of talking about an issue on his mind without triggering the counsellor to break client confidentiality. He was deflecting. In hindsight, Hawe's frequent desire to raise the issue of suicide was disturbing.

The notes from the 31 May session report that 'Alan very ashamed about porn/masturbation. Tried on Clodagh's underwear. Magazines. Caught red-handed. Bad piano results.'

'Tried on Clodagh's underwear.' Those words stopped me in my tracks. I thought of Clodagh and the stranger she lived with. She had no idea who he was or what he was capable of. Nobody did.

The garda notes said they asked the counsellor what 'caught red-handed' referred to. They noted that the counsellor 'didn't know' what Alan Hawe had been caught doing or where. They wrote: 'It may have been Clodagh that caught him red-handed, but [the counsellor] was not sure on this.' We don't believe Clodagh ever caught him 'red-handed'.

Clodagh was already upset about her husband continually looking at porn even though she had begged him to stop.

She confided in Mam that he refused to go to an addiction treatment centre such as the Rutland because he was afraid someone in the parish or the school would find out. She also told Mam she warned Hawe she would leave him if he didn't seek help. She confided everything to Mam.

I know she would have walked out on him and never returned if she knew what was really happening. We know now their marriage was hanging by a thread. If she had caught him 'red-handed' doing anything, it would have been the last straw for her.

Alan Hawe agreed to go to counselling to lull Clodagh into a false sense of security about getting 'help' for his porn issues. Clodagh was relieved because she thought he was dealing with their problems in a responsible and mature manner. She had no idea of the lies he was spinning around her.

She thought that Ryan and the wet floor had triggered all the upset at the school. But I believed Alan exaggerated that issue as a distraction from whatever real commotion was going on. After reading the counsellor's notes, I became even more convinced that the real reason behind his problems at school was because Hawe was 'caught red-handed' there. The counsellor seemed to confirm this when he later disclosed to gardaí: 'Alan masturbated somewhere he shouldn't have – possibly school.'

On 21 June 2016, the counsellor wrote: 'Alan had a really tough two weeks after [a colleague] and his school turned on him and accused him of bullying and intimidating her. Alan has attempted to talk to [this colleague] but met with "Baltic" response. Alan was afraid grievance coming. Very stressed.'

That was the last of Hawe's counselling sessions. Despite his recommendation that Hawe attend more sessions, the counsellor confirmed that he did not return after that date.

Even though Hawe attended counselling for his porn issues, he successfully downplayed his obsession. In the end, the counsellor told gardaí that Hawe was 'not addicted to porn'. There were gaps in the notes, many phrases that needed explaining and issues that should have been teased out.

As we pored over his session notes, we weren't aware that the investigation team had never interviewed the counsellor. They accepted a prepared statement from him eight months after the murders. I still find it incredible that it took eight whole months to collect a prepared statement from someone who should have been central to the investigation.

Even though the notes were only jottings, they provided new insights into the real Alan Hawe and what was going on in the months before the murders. They allowed a disturbing glimpse into the inner workings of his mind. Possibly masturbating in a school and putting on Clodagh's underwear revealed a more depraved side to the man than I ever thought possible. Yet, we were only barely grazing the depths of his darkness.

16

Anniversary Mass

Mam and I organised a first anniversary mass for Clodagh, Liam, Niall and Ryan on Sunday, 27 August 2017. We didn't ask Father Kelly to officiate for obvious reasons, liaising instead with another priest in the parish.

The week before, I left Mam at the graves and went into the church porch to pick up the parish newsletter. I wanted to see whether the anniversary mass was mentioned. Sure enough, it was listed, but just below it there was a listing for another anniversary mass – for Alan Hawe. That was the first time I'd heard about it, scheduled days later on Wednesday, 30 August.

My hand shook as I brought that leaflet to Mam, tending her daughter's and grandsons' graves. Three months had passed since Alan Hawe's body had been exhumed and moved out of the parish. Yet Father Kelly was marking the murderer's memory in the church mere metres from where his murder victims were laid to rest.

We were devastated. There was no need for that mass, considering Hawe's remains now lay elsewhere in the country. It showed so much disrespect to Clodagh and the boys. To us, it was like spitting on their graves.

In the year since Clodagh's murder, I'd learnt more about coercive control and domestic violence. Mam and I desperately wanted to see something positive come out of the horror that had happened to our family. We decided to raise money for other women and families at risk and do it in Clodagh and the boys' names.

More than fifty people attended our first committee meeting in St Joseph's Hall in Ballyjamesduff on 24 March 2017. We discussed setting up Cavan Lighthouse, a refuge for local families experiencing domestic violence in memory of Clodagh, Liam, Niall and Ryan. By the end of the meeting, our first fundraising campaign was arranged for the VHI Women's Mini Marathon at the start of June.

After a series of sales and events, we raised €44,122.92 but had to cease fundraising due to restrictions imposed by the charity regulator. Among other issues, meeting all the regulations imposed on a registered charity is a full-time job, and I had to earn a living. We decided to donate the funds to Tearmann Domestic Violence Service, a registered and respected charity in Cavan and Monaghan. In 2020 they opened a bank account in Clodagh, Liam, Niall and Ryan's names. We received six-monthly statements showing how the funds were used to pay for women's legal representation, food, clothes, and even Christmas presents for children. Tearmann has since merged with Safe Ireland, and this national charity is still in contact about where the funds are being directed.

Father Kelly's move to celebrate mass for a man who had murdered his family came as a particularly sickening blow, especially when I was immersed in fundraising for a women's refuge.

Mam and I knew there was little point in appealing to the priest's sense of decency. I still think it was a deliberate strike at us, two women who had dared to question his authority in the parish. He would never forgive us for making him use the word 'evil' in the context of his close friend.

We met with his bishop, Dr Leo O'Reilly, to appeal to him. But it was clear the ranks of the clergy were closed. 'I'm not going to tell Father Kelly what to do,' he said. He could not be persuaded to stop the mass.

I couldn't believe the indifference to the wishes of the victims' family. But we had to accept it – we could do nothing to stop the anniversary mass for Alan Hawe in Castlerahan church.

Instead, Mam and I and a small number of family members and friends held a quiet vigil at Clodagh and the boys' graves on the evening of the mass. Alan Hawe's parents were among those who attended the service. Another thirty locals, some of whom had sympathised with us at the time of the murders, were also there. People said afterwards, 'Well, only a few handfuls of people attended the mass,' but it was thirty people too many for us.

Whether they attended for Alan Hawe or as supporters of Father Kelly, I'll never know. But their presence told me that what Alan Hawe did was excusable in their eyes. I didn't care whether they held anniversary masses for him anywhere else in the country, but it was unforgivable to have a service in memory of a mass murderer next to where his victims were buried.

It seemed to me to highlight the church's lack of compassion, care or sensitivity towards women and other victims of male violence in our society.

17

The Murder Letter

Mam and I waited until Gary was in bed, and then we turned off the TV and our phones. In the quiet of my sitting room that December night, we read and reread the letter Alan Hawe had written on the night he'd murdered my sister and three nephews.

For sixteen months, the garda investigation team had ignored all our requests to see the letter. Detectives drip-fed us with a few excerpts but refused to let us read it. We kept being told it was evidence, even though there was no trial.

Mam and I were in our solicitor Liam Keane's office, in Dunshaughlin in Meath, that evening to work on the upcoming inquest. Liam was in the middle of itemising the documents he'd received when I heard something that made my heart skip a beat.

'You have Alan Hawe's murder letter?' I said, interrupting him. 'Can I see it?'

We never referred to this letter as a suicide note. Hawe committed four killings before he took his own life, so it has always been a murder letter to us.

The solicitor was astonished. 'It was addressed to you, and you haven't read it already?'

He copied the pages, and I stuffed them into my handbag, half relieved to have the letter and half in dread of reading what it contained. Hawe's bloodied fingerprints were found on the envelope and the front page, so the investigation team knew he had written it after the killings.

I'm not going to publish the entirety of Alan Hawe's murder letter in this book because it's almost wholly a list of self-absorbed, egotistical excuses and lies for why he decided it was best to murder his family. It also refers to people he knew in his past who may not want their names associated with it.

He said he'd thought about killing himself and staging it as an accident but feared he might be unsuccessful, and Clodagh would end up looking after him 'or, worse, knowing the truth'.

The letter contained a lot about why he felt he had no choice but to kill everyone.

'I know that Clodagh and the boys would never be able to live their hopes and dreams if I had killed myself. I know I would only be sentencing Clodagh to a life of misery.' He wrote, 'I also didn't want them to be thought of less by people just cos of the way their father was,' and 'I have to do this. I can't leave the boys orphans.'

Alan Hawe wanted us to believe that he'd thought only of their welfare and had done Clodagh and the boys a favour when he murdered them.

The letter was full of lies and red herrings. Knowing that his phone and computers would be examined in the investigation, Hawe used the following excuses to explain the sleaze they would discover in his browser history.

Sometimes recently when converting videos on ClipConverter, the odd dodgy website would pop up. I wasn't looking for this to happen and they were always blocked by the filter. I even looked at porn in the last few days on my phone but I knew I had cracked up and it helped me forget.

At two points in Hawe's letter, he also directed us to where we could find more information: 'Please contact ... the counsellor,' and 'The counsellor knows the rest,' he wrote.

The counsellor's notes provided a brief glimpse into the ten hours he spent listening to the inner thoughts of Alan Hawe. By then, our solicitor had also given us a copy of the prepared statement the counsellor had given to the gardaí.

But the prepared statement didn't tell us the rest. Indeed, that statement, handed over eight months after the murders, contained nothing that enlightened us further. Instead it was a polished document, professional in tone, containing condolences to the families, with a description of the counsellor's qualifications and his 'person-centred' approach to therapy.

The statement declared: 'There were no disclosures of a nature that would require confidentiality to be broken and a report made to other parties.' It added: 'In particular, there were no disclosures of physical violence and no disclosures of any harm to children. In our third counselling session, I asked Alan if he had any suicidal thoughts, and he said no.'

Of course Hawe lied all the time and admitted it in the following lines of his murder letter: 'They never knew the real me ... I just don't know what it was that I was so normal yet so dark and no one could see it.'

Hawe's condescending and patronising attitude towards Clodagh also stood out in his letter. 'Clodagh was the best ever,' and 'the boys were super', he wrote. 'They have a super mother and she has super boys.' My mother winced as she read that she, Mary, 'was super' too.

I shook my head in disbelief when I read Hawe's advice to his brother and me not to 'fuck up' our lives or our families' lives. His tone was one of superiority and condescension throughout. He knew better than all of us.

I read two lines over and over, hoping they didn't mean what I thought they meant, but I can't interpret them any other way: Alan Hawe said he enjoyed killing his family.

I think there was some sort of psychosis that made me enjoy that yet in the next moment I was the complete opposite. I'm sorry for how I murdered them all but I simply had no other way.

Or was that word 'psychosis' meant to spoonfeed the forensic psychologists with the suggestion that he had lost his mind? Any notion that he could have temporarily lost his mind was contradicted by the detailed list of instructions he wrote on a separate leaf. 'Please get Clodagh's jewellery on the bed and give it to Mary,' he wrote. He said to tell his brother 'to sell the car jeep'. There were other orders such as, 'Save our photos in the cabinet in the kitchen'; 'Tell the neighbours I'm sorry' and 'Get Clodagh's handbag on the clothes horse.' He was still trying to control everything from beyond the grave.

After killing his entire family, he also took time to write about the boys' credit union accounts and their money boxes. He noted that there was 'money in the Cadbury's Roses tin in the cabinet for the football club'. He left files full of financial documents on the kitchen table. Everything was organised, and no detail was missed.

The murder letter spans nearly a thousand words and refers to 'I' and 'me' 118 times. I don't believe it warrants any more paper than it already has. Most of it served to tell the reader how important he was to Clodagh and the boys and why he couldn't just kill himself and leave them behind.

But there are a few instances in which Alan Hawe may have revealed the real truth behind what happened that night. What jumped out at me immediately was the line 'I dreaded going back to school as it was all going to blow up.' He added, 'I just couldn't up and leave here either. The truth would have come out probably sometime.' Whatever the 'truth' was, he said, 'Clodagh and I were never going to come back from this, and I was leaving some mess for her to clean up.'

His letter suggested everything I suspected – that he was avoiding the consequences of something he had done at work. Whatever those secrets were, he didn't want Clodagh to know about them – another sure sign my sister hadn't been the one who had caught him 'red-handed'.

He feared Clodagh was about to find out what he had done and believed his life would unravel because these dark secrets were about to be exposed. Clodagh told our mother that she had been firm with Hawe: he had to sort out his issues with pornography and go to counselling. She said she would leave him if he didn't. He feared Clodagh was about to hear something that would prompt her to leave him for good. Had that fear triggered the murder spree?

But we were still in the dark. The investigators said they found no answers at the school despite initially saying what had happened there was 'the catalyst' to the murders. Clodagh had told us Hawe rang the teachers' union, the INTO. We wanted to know why he had called the union, whether for a grievance or to seek representation. If the gardaí had followed this up, they hadn't told us about it.

Hawe had also told Clodagh he'd seen an envelope with his name on it in a school filing cabinet. He was concerned about its contents. We didn't know what had become of it or whether the investigation had even requested it.

If Hawe's murder letter revealed anything, it was that it was no coincidence that he murdered his family on the night before he was due to meet with the staff on the first day back after the summer break. To this day, I believe something had happened at the school before the holidays that caused the dark events of that night.

That wintry night after Mam went home, I read and reread Hawe's words. They brought me to a very dark and lonely place. I was trembling and jumpy when I eventually shoved the letter into the back of a drawer. I remember hovering outside Gary's bedroom, almost frightened to open the door in case I found him like Hawe had left his three boys. For weeks after, I jumped at my own shadow and was scared of every noise. I knew I shouldn't, but I kept pulling out that letter and rereading it, trying to figure out what some of it meant.

For a long time, I had visualised Hawe sitting at the kitchen table, scribbling in black biro on sheets of A4 copier paper from their printer. I'd always assumed the letter was written in the kitchen, probably because it was left on the table with the folders containing all their financial details.

But investigations later confirmed that he had written it on the coffee-table, sitting on the couch beside Clodagh's bloodied remains.

As hard as I try to forget that letter now, those sick and twisted words and the chilling image of him writing it next to my dead sister continue to haunt me.

18

Stress

The county coroner, Dr Mary Flanagan, rang me one evening. It was her role to investigate the deaths of Clodagh, her boys and their murderer.

'Are you okay with the date of the inquest?' she asked.

At this stage, the inquest had been delayed for many months. We had expected it in the spring of 2017, but then Deputy State Pathologist Dr Michael Curtis had found traces of Hashimoto thyroiditis in Alan Hawe's post-mortem.

This discovery prompted Dr Flanagan and the gardaí to ask Professor Harry Kennedy, then the director of the Central Mental Hospital in Dundrum, to assess Hawe's mental state and whether he was psychotic during the murders. As a result, the inquest had to be pushed back to allow Professor Kennedy to complete his report.

We waited month after month, not knowing when it would happen. Finally, sometime in October, we heard the inquest was set for Monday, 18 December. It was difficult having so many unanswered questions for so long, and the delay was stressful, aggravating the grieving process, so I was anxious to get it over with.

I was confused by Dr Flanagan asking if I was okay with the inquest date. Mam and I would have preferred it to happen many months earlier.

'Well, yes, we're prepared for it,' I said. Mam and I had spent countless hours with our then new solicitor Liam Keane & Partners in Dunshaughlin.

'It's been on our minds for a long time now,' I added. 'Why are you asking?'

Dr Flanagan hesitated. 'I received a call from the parish priest of Castlerahan and another from a local TD asking for the date of the inquest to be changed. They said it is too near Christmas and doesn't suit the community. I didn't know whether you felt this way too.'

I couldn't believe what I was hearing. 'Dr Flanagan, we don't want any more delays,' I said. 'We want this inquest to go ahead as scheduled. We don't need it hanging over our heads any longer.'

I was livid when I got off the phone. Nothing surprised me where Father Kelly was concerned, but I was appalled that a public representative would try to influence the workings of the coroner's court. It didn't take long to discover the identity of this TD. The same TD had never contacted Mam or me to offer any assistance or advice after the murders. I rang him immediately.

'My mother and I have been waiting sixteen months for this inquest into the murders of four members of our family,' I said. 'We have a path worn driving fifty kilometres several nights a week to our solicitor's office trying to prepare for it. And neither of us can sleep with the stress of it. In the meantime, I'm trying to hold down a full-time job and prepare a normal, happy Christmas for my child. But you want this inquest postponed because you think a murder inquiry looks bad at Christmas? Let me make this clear – this inquest is going ahead whether you like it or not!'

I got a lot off my chest in that phone call, but the pre-inquest period was extremely stressful. The gardaí still did not furnish us with any information, and we were shocked when our solicitor gave us details of Professor Kennedy's report and the findings he would present to the inquest.

After reviewing Hawe's murder letter, GP records, and the counsellor's notes, Professor Kennedy said he believed Hawe was suffering from a severe mental illness and had psychotic episodes that had left his judgement 'severely impaired'. He concluded that Hawe had suffered from depression for years, maybe for a decade, which progressed to a more severe depressive episode and escalated until the murder-suicide.

I was stunned. 'Depression? God almighty. Alan Hawe

never suffered from depression in his entire life. I'm more depressed than Alan Hawe ever was.'

His GP of many years hadn't diagnosed depression; neither had his counsellor. None of his family ever saw evidence of it. I also believe Professor Kennedy's conclusions were an insult to people who suffer from depression yet don't go around murdering their families.

'We want to refute this evidence at the inquest,' I told the solicitor.

Our solicitor was hesitant as he addressed Mam and me. 'To do that, we'll have to seek independent expert opinion from a forensic psychiatrist or another expert in the UK.' He met our gaze, looking from one to the other of us. 'And you must be aware that this will delay the inquest further and involve thousands in costs and expenses.'

Mam and I exchanged a glance, deflated. The costs involved thousands of euros we did not have. My mother was already funding the solicitor for the inquest. We were acutely aware of the mounting legal fees.

'Even if we managed to secure independent expert medical evidence, its admissibility would be at the coroner's discretion,' he said.

I sighed. 'So, even if we managed to pay out all this money, we might not even be able to present it to the inquest?'

'That's it, I'm afraid.'

We had been told all along that the scope of an inquest was limited. In the event of sudden, unnatural, unexplained or violent death, an inquest's purpose is to ascertain the deceased's identity, when they died, where they died and how they died. These facts are called the 'who, what, where, when and how' of death. The reasons behind the deaths and the 'why' are not part of the inquest. The gardaí, solicitors, everyone warned us that 'why' my sister and nephews died was beyond the remit of the Coroners Act.

Yet the state had hired Professor Harry Kennedy to ascertain the 'why', and he had decided they were killed because Alan Hawe suffered from a severe depressive illness.

We asked whether we could put questions to Professor Kennedy at the inquest. No, we couldn't. If we did, the inquest would be adjourned. It felt like more silencing, more control. The guards would tell us nothing. We couldn't question anyone at the inquest. Our solicitor could ask questions on our behalf but couldn't interrogate witnesses.

The inquest, just like the whole investigation leading up to it, was hugely frustrating. All we wanted was a complete and thorough examination of the circumstances in which Clodagh, Liam, Niall and Ryan had died. For months now, we had had reason to doubt the thoroughness of the garda investigation into the deaths. Now the state seemed to have predetermined the inquest's verdict. Even worse, there was no one to whom we could voice our concerns. Mam and I were facing a brick wall every way we turned.

1 9

Inquest

My heart hammered as we walked through the cast-iron gates and across the tarmac car park of Cavan courthouse for the first day of the inquest. The courthouse is an imposing old building set back off Farnham Street, and walking up those granite steps under its vast portico is a daunting enough experience. But it was even more intimidating to approach it in the face of an enormous media presence. The rapid bursts of camera shutters surrounded us as we hurried along, and the media surged around us on the steps. It was terrifying.

My hollowed cheeks and the dark shadows under my eyes were evidence of my exhaustion. My sleep was poor, and the stress of the upcoming inquest had triggered my eating disorder again. Undereating and over-exercising were my coping mechanisms for dealing with emotional distress, trying to seize control of my body when other aspects of my life felt uncontrollable. Mam and I were also worn out from the preparations and driving to and from the solicitor's office every night after work.

And that courthouse held nothing but bad memories for us. As we entered the enormous entrance hall and followed our solicitor, I realised we were heading for the same room used for Tadhg's inquest six years earlier, courtroom number two.

Even though I had pushed for the inquest to begin, I dreaded it. I'd been through this traumatic process twice before with Tadhg and then Richie, so I didn't enter that room with any illusions. The requirements of the Coroners Act are quite restrictive, and I knew many avenues would remain unexplored. It is a court of inquiry, a public fact-finding hearing rather than a trial, so there is no prosecution or defence. But I never expected the process to leave so many questions unanswered.

The room was small and packed to its capacity of forty or fifty people. The coroner was at the top of the room, and immediately below her were the solicitors representing the Hawes' and our legal teams sitting at separate tables. Mam and I sat in the rows behind them with Gerry, Carmel, Melissa and Audrey. I recognised some friendly faces, including Clodagh's teaching colleagues from Oristown. The seven jury members sat immediately to my left, close to a gallery of seats set aside for gardaí and other witnesses. The media sat in a gallery ahead to my right. I didn't see a sign of the Hawes that morning, and I believe they never attended the two-day inquest.

The coroner, Dr Mary Flanagan, was a trim, middle-aged woman with short sandy hair and a no-nonsense approach. Coroners are either qualified solicitors or medical practitioners appointed by local authorities. Like many coroners, Dr Flanagan was a full-time GP.

In her opening comments, she said this would be a 'particularly emotive' inquest that would last at least two days and involve evidence from more than a dozen witnesses.

Mam was the first to take the stand to deliver an account of the morning of 29 August 2016. It was a nerve-racking ordeal for her, and I'll never forget how fragile she looked in the witness box. Her voice quivered when she swore the oath, her hand on the Bible, and she struggled to talk through her tears. Yet her composure in the face of overwhelming grief showed remarkable strength and conviction. Once again, I saw the resilience of a mother who had endured the unthinkable loss of two of her three children and three of her four grandsons. I don't know many women like her.

A guard read her statement to the court and, under everyone's gaze, Mam relived the day she lost four of her loved ones. She then answered some questions from the coroner, who was always kind and solicitous, but Mam was still ashen-faced and shattered when she returned to her seat.

Garda Alan Ratcliffe of Ballyjamesduff garda station gave evidence next, describing Mam as visibly upset when he arrived on the scene that morning. He said he had met her with Clodagh's next-door neighbour, Edie Harrigan. He told of how he had used one of Mam's keys to enter the house through the back door at 11.21 a.m., where he discovered all five bodies.

His colleague, Garda Aisling Walsh, became emotional as she described the moment when she saw the bodies of Liam and Niall. My heart went out to her, seeing her pause to collect herself before she recalled the horrific scene. I felt thankful again that Mam never saw what lay inside that house.

Several other guards gave evidence at that point. The Garda Technical Bureau gave depositions about forensics and further details from the scene. A handwriting expert spoke about finding Alan Hawe's murder letter and confirmed it was his writing. Evidence was given that they had identified the right palm print of Alan Hawe on the bloodstained hatchet and his murder letter. We heard Clodagh's DNA was found on the blade end of one weapon and Alan's Hawe's clothing. It was all technical, yet every detail was sickening for us. I flinched when one of the depositions mentioned finding a 'clump' of black hair in the hallway, as I knew it had to have been Clodagh's.

The inquest adjourned until the afternoon for the arrival of Deputy State Pathologist Dr Michael Curtis. The post-mortem evidence was far worse than we expected. Alan Hawe's savagery and deviousness were exposed in disturbing detail, and we learnt the full horror of the murders of Clodagh and her children for the first time. I remember Mam and I gripping each other's hands throughout his harrowing evidence.

Dr Flanagan asked Dr Curtis whether his investigations offered any insight into who had died first.

He replied he believed that Hawe had killed Clodagh and Liam initially, then Niall and Ryan. 'By dispatching Clodagh and the older boy first, he would have rendered the possibility of a physical challenge less likely,' he said.

It seemed like further evidence that this had been a cold and calculated assassination of his family rather than an explosive act of madness.

We heard Clodagh was found lying face down on the couch in the sitting room, wearing her blue polka-dot pyjamas and a purple dressing gown. We knew from the garda investigation that she had been looking at holiday destinations on her tablet that night. She was relaxing, having a cup of tea in a place where she was entitled to feel safe. The pathologist found considerable bloodstaining on the couch and the floor beneath her. The coffee-table in front of her was bloodstained, as were the tablet she was using, the TV remote control, her iPhone and her overturned mug.

The black-handled knife and axe he had used to kill her were found strewn to the left of the sofa. I felt ill as the pathologist reported he had found a deep wound in Clodagh's right hand, a defensive wound as she turned and tried to fend off Hawe and his axe or knife. I couldn't stop thinking of what Clodagh went through in those moments. The pathologist referred to fractures, axe blows, and stab wounds to the head, neck and body. Hawe killed Clodagh as if he hated her, murdering her with savagery. She died from axe puncture wounds to the head and neck.

Mam and I clenched each other's hands as his evidence brought to life the true brutality of the murders.

Dr Curtis told the hearing that he found it 'very difficult to believe that it's entirely coincidental that the boys suffered wounds below the Adam's apple' that would 'have rendered all three of them unable to make a sound'. We were shaken, sickened to our cores to learn how Hawe had killed them all. With clinical precision, he had cut their throats, preventing them from alerting each other or neighbours by crying out.

Just how much planning and research had Hawe put into these killings, I wondered. He had to have studied this. How else would he have known how to murder them in this manner?

After killing Clodagh, Hawe went up the stairs, took the first door on his right and entered Liam and Niall's bedroom.

Liam lay sleeping on the bed to the left as you came in the door. It was a warm August night, so he was only in underwear when Hawe used a knife to stab and slice his neck. My heart still breaks knowing that Liam woke during the process and died knowing what his father had done to him. We know this because the pathologist reported that he found two defensive stab wounds to Liam's right hand and scratches across his left forearm from the struggle. He desperately tried to defend himself.

Niall's bed was arranged end-to-end with his brother's. That summer night, he wore tartan pyjama bottoms. The pathologist observed that Niall had placed his spectacles on a pile of books on his bedside locker. I cried as I heard that Niall also struggled with his father's dark shadow that night. I tried not to imagine the terror he experienced before he died, but the pathologist found defensive stab wounds to his hands too. We heard that Hawe tossed duvets over the dead or dying boys before leaving their bedroom.

Hawe also suffered wounds to his forearms and hands, which Dr Curtis described as injuries from his victims.

Ryan was the last of the boys to die. They know this because the bloodied murder weapon, another black-handled knife like the one he had used on Clodagh, was abandoned on his pillow. Ryan was wearing wine and grey pyjamas and clutching his soft toy, Dreamy, when Hawe came for him with his blade.

The pathologist's words to describe Ryan's death will always haunt me and can never be unheard. He gave details I can't bear to relate.

A wordless wail emerged from deep inside me, and I couldn't contain the grief during this evidence. Mam was audibly upset now too. The room felt too hot and airless, and bile rose in my throat. The details of Ryan's death were overwhelmingly distressing, even on a day full of hideous revelations.

While we were still reeling from the post-mortem evidence, the pathologist reported finding traces of Hashimoto thyroiditis but gave evidence that Hawe's brain showed no evidence of intrinsic disease. The pathologist reported the murderer's body was discovered hanging from a banister pole in the front hall. He had used an orange nylon rope wound twice around his neck. There was no doubt he was the culprit. His hands were stained with Clodagh and the boys' blood, and scratches from his struggling victims were evident on both his hands.

The evidence was far more appalling than I expected, and I left that day feeling broken and re-traumatised. In truth, the grieving process began again and was even exacerbated by the experience. I didn't have to attend the inquest. I chose to listen to the post-mortem details because I needed to know how Clodagh and the boys had died.

But did our family have to be exposed to those revelations

for the first time in the full glare of the public and the media? Could they not have accorded us the dignity and respect of receiving this information about our loved ones behind closed doors? I'm thinking of many other families who will go through the same inquest process when I say there should be a better, kinder way.

20

Inquest Day 2

We ran the gauntlet of the media outside Cavan courthouse again the next day. I never got used to it. I appreciated the public's right to know what happened that night in Castlerahan and the lessons that could be learnt to save other vulnerable women. But Mam and I were not public figures, and neither of us wanted our faces, etched with grief, appearing on newspapers or TV news programmes. It was another added stress, another trauma and another unwelcome hurdle to negotiate each day.

The first witness on day two was the counsellor. We hoped to learn more about Hawe through his appearance at the inquest. However, his evidence essentially repeated what he had recorded in his garda statement. He noted that Hawe placed a lot of emphasis on being seen as a good husband and father and his good standing in the community.

He also said that on their third session together, he spoke to Hawe about suicide and that his client gave no indication of an intention to harm himself or anyone else. On the final session on 21 June 2016, he said Hawe wept as he told him, 'People think of me as a pillar of the community ...' before pausing to add '... If only they knew.'

The counsellor said he gave Hawe some coping mechanisms for stress over the summer holidays and never saw him again. Hawe's reasons for attending counselling were never really addressed in the courtroom, so there was no mention of his issues with pornography. Nor was there any reference to anything else raised in the sessions, such as cross-dressing. The counsellor's summation was that Alan Hawe 'had a fear of being seen as someone less than perfect'.

Even though Hawe's murder letter twice urged us to contact his counsellor to get 'the rest' of the information about him, this was not raised at the inquest. I really wanted to address the witness and pose some questions, but I stayed quiet. I was afraid. It had repeatedly been said that the inquest would be adjourned if we spoke up.

The coroner was kind and occasionally stopped to ask if we had any questions about the process. But the inquest did not allow for us to address any questions directly to the witnesses, much as we might have wanted to. We were not seated beside our solicitor, and so could not get him to intercede on our behalf.

Dr Paula McKevitt, Clodagh's family GP and mine, was called as the next witness. She said that Alan Hawe had attended her surgery in June 2016 for a sore toe. He had used bleach to treat the nail before coming to the surgery. She said he also expressed concerns over not sleeping, and felt run down with a sore throat and mouth ulcers.

She took bloods, and prescribed anti-fungal medication for his toe, and Stilnoct, a brand name for the sleeping drug zolpidem.

She also said he mentioned the family's upcoming trip to Italy. The doctor spoke about meeting Clodagh afterwards, and when she asked about the trip, she was told it was a 'good holiday'. The doctor didn't see a sign of 'delusional' behaviour during Hawe's visits. 'His behaviour seemed normal,' she said, adding: 'Nothing in the consultation ... suggested any despair or hopelessness. He appeared positive in his outlook at the time.'

The doctor also said she was unaware of any 'history of depression' in Hawe. Nor had he ever told her that he was attending counselling. 'He did not disclose any of his deep thoughts to me,' she said.

However, she stated that 'the [work] conflict prior to the summer recess was a great source of stress', adding, 'He was concerned about a conflict that had arisen with a colleague, and he reported feeling isolated as a result.'

The Central Mental Hospital's Professor Harry Kennedy was the next witness. Having read his report, we knew what his evidence would be to the inquest. He said he had conducted his psychiatric post-mortem based on the counsellor's notes, Alan Hawe's GP records and the contents of his murder letter. He stated his belief that long-standing depression, possibly ten years or more, and a 'severe depressive episode with psychotic symptoms' was probably the root cause of the murders.

Our solicitor, Liam Keane, was constrained within the remit of the inquest when questioning a witness. But he asked whether a person suffering a difficulty would consider their next action to be the 'destruction of their family'.

'I believe his judgement was severely impaired. That's what I believe happened in this case,' Professor Kennedy replied.

That was when Mam suddenly defied her silencers. She sat forward in her seat and addressed the psychiatrist, her voice ringing loud and clear in the room. Afterwards, she said she didn't know what came over her, but she thought it must have been Clodagh who prompted her to speak out. 'Do you never interview families?' she said.

The professor offered his condolences to the family, but Mam reiterated what she said. 'Did you consider when compiling this report interviewing families of the people who were murdered or the family of the murderer?'

Professor Kennedy didn't have the chance to reply as the coroner jumped to his defence. 'To be fair, he is my expert,' she said, adding he was presenting his expert opinion because she had asked him to review all documents and give his view. But Mam addressed the psychiatrist again, nonetheless.

'But my question is, seeing as you never met Alan Hawe, Clodagh or his family, did you ever consider speaking to the family in relation to how he was? I knew him for twenty years. I didn't know him, but I knew him.'

Professor Kennedy said something about being constrained in evidence before the coroner. And that was it. The inquest moved on, and any avenue of enquiry concerning the psychiatrist's report was closed.

I had questions too. I wondered why the coroner hadn't asked the psychiatrist to interview family members, relatives and friends. It's called a psychological autopsy. It can be a valuable part of an investigation into a suicide. Might the psychiatrist have come to an entirely different expert opinion if he had done that?

Alan Hawe's excellent family GP never saw a sign of depression in the five years she treated him. I wanted to ask the psychiatrist how he could explain that. Or could he explain how everyone in Hawe's family failed to detect this so-called 'long-standing' depression over the past ten years? In his murder letter, Hawe wrote, 'If it's any consolation, we were happy.' I wanted to ask whether he thought it was rare to hear someone suffering from depression say he was happy.

I also wanted to ask whether he thought someone experiencing a psychotic episode could plan murders months in advance, as Alan Hawe had done. And could he murder his family, then calmly go online, enter his bank passwords and PIN and transfer funds?

But the questions went unasked and unanswered. The victims' families do not have a voice in an inquest. They are muzzled, silenced and sidelined in the proceedings.

The coroner declined to release the contents of Alan Hawe's murder letter to the public courtroom but gave the jury access to the pages. And that was it, really.

By the end of that day, the jury returned verdicts of unlawful killing following the coroner's recommendation. I recall the jury forewoman's voice breaking with emotion when reading the verdict for Ryan.

The jury ruled Alan Hawe's death a suicide, which was also in line with the recommendation of the coroner. The Hawes' solicitor accepted the verdict.

At its heart, the purpose of an inquest is to use information discovered during the investigation to prevent further avoidable deaths. This is done by issuing recommendations along with the verdict. After reading Hawe's letter and hearing the evidence of the witnesses, the jury recommended that steps be taken to 'raise awareness of mental health issues at work'. It was clear to the jury that issues at work were important in this case.

There were five references to the school or specific people in the school scattered about Hawe's murder letter. 'I was not teaching properly'; 'The kids probably said I was on the phone or computer ...' More explicitly, he wrote, 'I dreaded going back to school as it was all going to blow up.' He murdered everyone on the night before he was due to return to school. The counsellor's deposition referred to his client's worries because of an incident at the school. Hawe's GP spoke of his concerns about a conflict with a colleague. Yet not a single person from Hawe's national school in Castlerahan was called as a witness to the inquiry.

The evident premeditation and calculated nature of the killings were never addressed either. The fact these murders were planned, possibly from the beginning of the summer holidays in June, was never mentioned in the entire inquest.

It felt so frustrating that none of these issues could be raised. We had many unanswered questions, and much of what we heard was lip service and sympathy. Mam and I were effectively gagged in this public inquiry into the murders of our loved ones. We were mere observers instead of integral to the process of investigating the tragedy.

To me, it seemed the authorities were determined to spin the psychiatrist's narrative of events: Alan Hawe, the devoted family man, snapped because of depression. It was a murder-suicide and family tragedy that couldn't have been avoided. Let's wrap this up and go home, case closed.

It was devastating. If the case were left like this, we felt that no lessons would ever be learnt from our family tragedy. With no insight into how and why this had happened, how many more murder-suicides would there be? How many more times would the authorities continue to wring their hands, say how awful it was, blame it on depression and move on?

I was reeling as we walked out from under the portico of Cavan courthouse. 'Reeling' is the only word I can think of to describe the mix of exhaustion, pain, despair and shock of those two days. I stood dazed with Mam behind our solicitor as he read out our statement afterwards. Mam and I had written it hastily; our solicitor reviewed and edited it.

On 29 August 2016, we lost our daughter and sister Clodagh and her lovely sons Liam, Niall and Ryan in the most horrific circumstances. They were savagely and brutally killed by Alan Hawe in a premeditated and calculated manner.

We are aware that the inquest has a limited role in law in that its function is restricted to establishing how, where and when our loved ones died. However, it is clear from the evidence presented that Clodagh and the boys were killed in a sequence that ensured that the eldest and most likely to provide effective resistance were killed first and that they were executed in a manner which rendered them unable to cry out for help.

The inquest does not address why Alan Hawe committed this savagery, but his counsellor has said that he was concerned about his position as 'a pillar of the community', and we are aware that he was concerned at his imminent fall from that position and the breakdown of his marriage.

While the psychiatrist has attempted as best he could to create a retrospective diagnosis based on items and records, his GP, who knew him for five years, said he never displayed any signs of depression ...

I hardly heard Liam Keane as he read out those words. Myself and Mam were almost overwhelmed with all the questions we wanted to ask and the issues we wanted to raise. We wanted to scream them from the rooftops.

A million emotions had been wrung out of me over those two long days, but I left the inquest crushed and disappointed that our quest to discover what really lay behind the events in that house in August 2016 was still being frustrated.

21

Lost Innocence

The final line of our inquest statement requesting the media 'to respect our privacy and allow us to grieve' fell upon deaf ears. Afterwards, Mam and I hurried down Cavan's main street in tears, heads down, with reporters and photographers in hot pursuit.

A car pulled alongside us, and someone shouted out the window: 'Leave those women alone!' A stranger could see our distress. I wasn't fit to talk, and what was there to say? I felt steamrolled by the process. We needed to retreat, recover and figure out what to do next.

I drove us to the graveyard at Castlerahan. I needed to soak up some of the peace and tranquillity of the leafy surroundings. I usually find a sense of perspective and clarity from being in the silence of the graveyard. I gazed at Clodagh and the boys' headstone with six little butterflies etched into the polished granite. Those striking Red Admirals continued to appear in our lives after Clodagh and the boys died, and we added six small butterfly engravings to the stone to represent them, Tadhg and Richie.

We were only in the graveyard a few minutes when I thought I heard something. I looked around. We were alone in the place.

'Mam, do you hear that?'

'What?'

'It sounds like a camera.'

I thought I could hear the same staccato burst of mechanical clicking that I'd heard outside the inquest. The sound was aggressive, almost predatory, but this time it seemed distant.

Mam glanced around and said I was paranoid.

I scanned around me again. We were the only people in the graveyard. 'Maybe you're right,' I said.

We walked further into the graveyard towards Richie's grave, and suddenly, something leapt from a tree in front of us. The man, previously concealed amid the branches, didn't spare a glance at our startled faces. He tore away, his camera held aloft, sprinting towards the cemetery wall. He sprang nimbly over it, and we heard his car tearing off before we could follow him.

Mam and I stood there stunned, hardly believing what we'd just witnessed. We couldn't even have the space and time to grieve. We felt laid bare that day.

The intense media interest since the murders made me feel even more anxious than I already felt. It made it harder to cope. I also had Gary to worry about. I was trying to protect him from what was going on.

The following day my heart pounded with shock when I went to the shops and saw the piles of newspapers. Two newspapers had printed a close-up of my face, slap, bang on their front pages. I had been crying, and my eyes were swollen and red. It felt so intrusive, being exposed by the cameras during one of the worst days of my life.

I didn't want Gary to see this. He was only four and a bright child. I didn't want him asking, 'Why is your face on the paper, and why are you crying?' I was afraid to bring him to the shops for days after. I was trying to keep as much as possible of what had been going on away from him.

He had to be told some of what had happened because he'd heard things at school and in the community. My psychologist Dr Paul Gaffney has been incredibly kind and has come to our house to help me answer Gary's questions. He advised I should use simple, clear language and be honest. He has always emphasised it's important to be truthful. He says to let Gary steer the conversation and the questions, and if I don't know the answers, it's okay to say so.

I'm so thankful to have Dr Gaffney's help and support. But sometimes Gary's questions are a stark reminder that everyone needs to be careful when discussing adult topics in front of children. They hear everything, absorb far more than we realise and regurgitate these things in the schoolyard. When it's not age-appropriate information, it can scar young lives.

Like any parent, I want to protect Gary and give him a normal, happy childhood. No parent should have to live in constant fear of what their child might hear before they're old enough to process it. If I had my way, he still wouldn't know about this. He is too young and innocent.

22

Therapy

Several senior managers sat on the other side of the desk, eyes steely, expressions stern. I regretted not bringing someone with me as soon as I set foot in the room. Earlier, I'd asked whether someone could accompany me for support, but they told me it wasn't that kind of meeting – it wasn't a disciplinary meeting.

I loved working as HR manager in Clontarf Hospital, but the mental strength required for a ninety-minute commute each way while being a single mum to a then three-year-old boy was too challenging to continue in the middle of a murder investigation. I took another role nearer home that was not in my career plan and while working for that organisation, an issue had arisen over my occupational health form. These forms are concerned with how work and the environment affect an employee's health and how their health can affect their ability to do their job.

Around the time of the inquest, an employee complained that my personal life was affecting their mental health. I had never shared my personal life with them; the examples given to management were what they had read in the news. I was stunned and hurt by this complaint but could do little about it.

No formal complaint had been lodged, so I never had the opportunity to respond. Instead, a verbal complaint had been made.

I was shocked when I received my occupational health form to read a note seeking advice on 'how [further court cases] may impact on Jacqueline and potentially other members of the team'. The managers believed I should agree to this and sign the form. But I was confused.

'My occupational health referral form should relate to me. The issue you're referring to has nothing to do with my health or my ability to do my work.'

But they continued telling me that I must sign this form. I became emotional. My anxiety spiralled, and my pulse raced. It seemed they were determined I was not leaving the room until I signed my consent. And then one of the panel leant in, eyes narrowed and said, 'Do you have some kind of impediment that you can't understand this?'

That was when I crumbled. I began messily sobbing, my shoulders heaving. Humiliated and overwrought, I just wanted to escape the room. I snatched the document, signed it against my will and left. I never returned to that place of work.

I had worked hard to recover after what had happened to my husband, my sister and nephews. I had completed my post-grad when I was four months pregnant, four weeks after my husband died, and I had come in the top five percentile of the class.

But being asked if I had 'an impediment' shattered my confidence. Alan Hawe was not even related to me, yet I felt I was being punished for what he had done. Management supported a colleague who complained that their mental health was affected by what had happened to my family.

That night I was distraught. I reasoned that if all these senior managers with a background in HR agreed with the complainant, perhaps they were right. Maybe I *was* stupid. I couldn't keep a job or earn a living, so what was the point in continuing? It felt hopeless. I thought Gary and Mam would be better off without me, and I wrote suicide letters to both that night.

The strange thing is that until that meeting I'd thought I was doing well. Immediately after the murders, I'd started seeing a psychologist. I got a new job closer to home, so I didn't have the long motorway commute to Dublin. I was coping and trying to do all the right things for my health. I didn't realise then that trauma, especially cumulative traumas, has a way of sneaking up on you.

After surviving everything that had happened before, it seemed unbelievable that I would fall to my knees because I was accused of having 'an impediment'. I was vulnerable and didn't realise it.

Dr Paul Gaffney:

For Jacqueline, that work incident was the straw that broke the camel's back. A breakdown often happens like that. There's a concern or something that causes distress that seems almost incidental compared with all the real traumas that occurred in the past.

However, any one incident can exacerbate all the other awful things that happened. Experiencing so much trauma in her life meant Jacqueline was in a lot of pain. When you're in that much pain, you either go through periods where you're incredibly numb, where you don't feel or can't feel anything, or periods where you're incredibly sensitive.

It's not a great metaphor, but trauma is like having sore teeth. Everything hurts, hot tea, cold water, and there's no respite. Trauma had left Jacqueline with no emotional skin. She felt raw, so any unkindness or negative comment seeped through and wounded her far more deeply than someone who hadn't experienced trauma.

She felt intense physical pain because trauma is a physical experience. It's horrible, and it's scary. It's also very weird for the person experiencing it. For most people who have been traumatised, it's a painful, physical experience.

They can feel like an open wound. What happened in the workplace that day was a trauma too much for Jacqueline.

I didn't have time to do anything stupid that night because Mam came along at the right time. I broke down and told her everything, and she gave me the support to keep going and get help. I remember sitting at Mam's kitchen table days later, my head in my hands. The psychologist I'd been seeing for the previous two years said I needed more help than she could give me. She said she was referring me to another psychologist who had experience in treating trauma. I felt complete despair.

'What is the point in this? What is the point in seeing another psychologist?' I cried. 'He's going to nod and smile and listen, but he won't be able to help me.'

Dr Paul Gaffney:
In March 2018, I began seeing Jacqueline, after I was appointed Senior Psychologist to Cavan primary care in 2017. The murders of Clodagh and her children had a profound impact in Cavan. It was like the world ended – a 9/11-type moment. I met Jacqueline through one of my former colleagues, Dr Aedamar Bergin. Aedamar had built up a relationship with Jacqueline, but by March 2018, she realised that Jacqueline needed more help and needed to be seen more frequently.

'You've more trauma experience because most of your career has been working with trauma, so I think you would be a good fit with Jacqueline,' she said. 'Would you look after her?'

She made it clear that this would be a special assignment, very different from most other primary care psychology cases.

Jacqueline and I began with a few phone calls, and then I remember the initial meeting in April 2018. I had a new colleague that day, Aisling Hagerty, an assistant psychologist, and we both met Jacqueline that Friday evening in Virginia, around 5.30 p.m., after the regular clinic was over.

For the first year and several months, we both worked with Jacqueline. Then Aisling moved on, and I continued.

I went to see Paul on 6 April 2018 – I remember the date because it was Richie's anniversary. Paul's new assistant psychologist, Aisling, was with him. I went into that room pessimistic and despairing, not expecting this to go anywhere.

But Paul's brand of care was completely different from that of any therapist before. He's a solution-focused therapist. I was on sick leave and told him what had happened at work, and his immediate reaction was, 'Well, this is not going to continue.'

He said he'd write to the organisation and explain my psychological needs. He said they had a duty of care to provide a safe space and a safe working environment. I felt a ray of hope again, and it all started to snowball from that day.

Dr Paul Gaffney:

From the start, I knew there was something special about this woman because she was remarkable to be standing at all. At that moment, work was the pressing issue for Jacqueline.

She was out of work on sick leave, which was not a good thing after suffering the traumas Jacqueline had been through. And her work situation was exacerbating all the other terrible things that had happened to her.

My focus was, 'Okay, we need to sort this out before touching all that other trauma.' I remember Jacqueline looking at me as if to say, 'Okay, well, how do we do that?' She'll be the first to admit that she had no expectations of that meeting. I suggested I write to the head of HR and explain how Jacqueline had been through a horrific deal of trauma and was now at home on sick leave because she didn't feel safe or supported at work.

I was very aware that when people come to a psychologist or therapist, the critical question is, can I trust this person? Is this person dependable? By committing to writing this letter, I had helped her see me as trustworthy, as someone who wanted to help. She had been invalidated at work, and we took that on board, advocated for her and went from there.

And I think she also liked having both Aisling and me as therapists. For Jacqueline, it was like being heard twice.

Paul taught me that I had all the symptoms of what is known as vicarious trauma – that I had been traumatised by indirect exposure to traumatic events. Those symptoms can include feelings of grief, anxiety, sadness, nightmares, irritability and anger. Sufferers can also feel isolated and unsafe.

Paul also diagnosed me with post-traumatic stress disorder (PTSD). I was jumpy when it came to sudden noises, and I still am. That never goes away. My colleagues at work often laughed at my visible reaction when someone came up behind me or slammed a door. One manager was always careful to cough gently when he was behind me because otherwise I leapt with fright. Most people found it hilarious, and I always felt stupid for overreacting. But I still tremble after any loud or sudden noise.

I also had a lot of distressing flashbacks from the day I found Richie. I was frequently overwhelmed with intrusive thoughts about Clodagh and the boys' deaths. I didn't know these were symptoms of PTSD and that I was constantly in a state of alarm and hypervigilance. I learnt that I had probably suffered from PTSD since the day I'd found Richie.

Dr Paul Gaffney:

At its simplest, the human brain is essentially almost three million years old. The part of the brain that deals with trauma is a fist-size area at the top of the spinal cord called the amygdala. Essentially, it's an alarm box, and the problem with alarm boxes is that there are only two settings – on and off.

Even though our species has evolved, we are basically still wired for survival. The amygdala was useful in days when there might be a dinosaur around every corner or a rival tribe over the hill. When people talk about having a sixth sense that something's not quite right, that's the amygdala at work. The amygdala is one of the reasons that we're still here on the planet when other species aren't. So, that's the good news.

The bad news is that when it's triggered, the amygdala responds to everything as if it's life and death. For example, if you narrowly avert a car crash, you will often have a flash of fear, anger, or an intense emotion rush through your body seconds later. Nothing happened, but you can experience extreme anxiety or anger. This is the amygdala reacting to the threat, and that feeling may arise again when you sit back in the car next time. The amygdala is again warning of the danger of being in a car.

The problem with the amygdala is it's a one-gear solution to threat. There's either danger or no danger. Jacqueline suffered vicarious trauma rather than trauma because she wasn't assaulted herself. But there's very little difference between the two because when she thinks about the awful things that happened to Clodagh and the boys, the brain does not distinguish between it happening to her or Clodagh. The brain perceives it as a threat, a constant danger to Jacqueline too, and the amygdala is on full alert.

Successive traumas mean that the brain is always switched on and alert for risk. The person is hyperaroused and hypervigilant, and it's a very physical feeling.

Paul started treating me with cognitive behavioural therapy (CBT) and eye movement desensitisation and reprocessing (EMDR), a treatment designed to reduce the distress associated with traumatic memories.

Paul would talk me through the experience of finding Richie, minute by minute, for example. I started remembering more by continually going through these events, and the images and memories increasingly lost their power over me. The EMDR made me stronger.

Dr Paul Gaffney:

I believe to be an effective therapist, you need old-fashioned empathy, kindness, thoughtfulness, and the ability to walk in someone's shoes. That's a lot of the journey in therapy, but there are also ways of treating trauma.

I'm trained in a specific trauma approach called EMDR. Most traumas hold power over us even if we're not conscious of it or unsure what the trauma is. The brain is incredibly sophisticated and often won't let you remember the worst of what happened, whereas the body remembers everything.

Often, the person can't discern any conscious reason for feeling fearful, scared, anxious or why they have that sixth sense that something terrible will happen.

The Body Keeps the Score *by Bessel van der Kolk is the pre-eminent text in this work. Traumatised people experience awful, overwhelming physical feelings but often have no conscious explanation or memories of what these feelings are about.*

What EMDR does is help a person process those feelings and bring them into consciousness within the realm of a safe relationship. I was very sceptical until I did the training when I was working with traumatised children who often didn't have the words to describe what had happened.

We ask the patient to follow a pen or finger to stimulate eye movement from side to side and grab the brain's attention. If we do this at speed, it can help people process scary feelings, and if we do it slowly, this rocking motion can help people install images or mantras that help them feel safer. It sounds bizarre and, like many things in psychology, we're not quite sure how it works, but the research is compelling.

So, we started to help Jacqueline by getting her to process the story, particularly the events surrounding Clodagh and the boys. The awful thing with trauma is that every additional trauma makes the previous trauma seem more significant and powerful. There was so much trauma in Jacqueline's case that it was almost overwhelming.

Paul's methods worked for me. Instead of sitting there and telling him and Aisling what had upset me, they responded. They came up with ideas about possible solutions and what they might look like.

Paul would say, 'What might happen to you, Jacqueline, if you did A, B or C?' Paul geared me up for every conversation or confrontation I faced, and we discussed how best to handle it. What sometimes looked like a huge issue when I arrived for a session was much reduced by the time I left.

Dr Paul Gaffney:
We did two things. First, we validated Jacqueline. We worked very hard to help her see that she was right to feel upset, she was right to be annoyed, and her feelings were valid and understandable. Everything hurts when you're in a lot of psychological pain like Jacqueline was.

So, some days, she would come in, and she wouldn't talk about the murder of her sister at all. Instead, she spoke about something that to the average person might seem incidental: a phone call not returned, a hurtful remark, an unkind deed. But because of Jacqueline's pain, anything could become an additional heartbreak.

The transformation in me wasn't overnight. After the initial feeling of relief, I soon felt very low again. Mostly, it was because the work situation took a long time to be sorted out.

So, for a long time, I felt hopeless. I spent eight months on sick leave, feeling unwanted and useless. And what made it worse was this was all over a situation that I couldn't control. The trouble at work had started because of what Alan Hawe had done. I worried that the sick pay would end too, so I felt a lot of stress that year.

Dr Paul Gaffney:

We hit a very dark period in August 2018 when Jacqueline was suicidal. She reached a time when she was no longer hopeful. That was a couple of months into it. It's almost as if there was an initial high because she felt someone understood her. Then everything plunged again.

The enormity of what happened and the awfulness of what happened hit her, and that awful darkness and blackness took over. We were still trying to clarify the work situation and advocate for Jacqueline, sometimes even trying to ensure she got paid. We were still trying to find a new post for her. Meanwhile, she felt nobody wanted her because of what had happened.

The biggest fear in my job is somebody kills themselves on our watch. It's the thing you worry most about. The good thing about Jacqueline was that she never stopped engaging and never stopped trying. She has incredible courage. Unearthing traumatic emotions and buried memories can be frightening. Sometimes, this work gets too painful, and the therapist represents all the pain, so people don't want to talk to you for a while. Jacqueline never stopped talking. She has tremendous strength.

At one point, she said, 'Paul, will this get any better?'

And I said, 'Well, there are no guarantees it will.'

'What do I need to do?' she asked.

'Well, apart from doing what you're doing, we have to help you find some meaning here and create something positive from this.'

So, Jacqueline decided that she would make a difference, make a change, and that was when she discovered her internal strength. She began seeing how she could make a difference and find meaning from what happened.

Jacqueline started to see that the story must be told. She threw off the sense of shame and stigma she associated with the murders and started telling her truth and her story. Much of her story was never uttered before she spoke about it in therapy. Once Jacqueline was able to talk about it in therapy, she was able to tell everyone.

But if someone had spoken to her about it in early 2018, she wouldn't have remembered much of the story because it would have been too awful. When Jacqueline recalled her past, it would have overwhelmed her. She got used to talking about these things in the safe place we provided. It was almost as if she was in rehearsals for the interviews that followed.

That has been hugely significant. By the time she went public in 2019, there had been an enormous transformation. And once she went out there and told her story, that changed everything.

Only for Paul and Aisling, I believe I wouldn't be here now. They turned everything around for me and remain close friends even now. Paul has always supported me and given me solutions to issues that arise. And that has built up my resilience.

More than anything, he has helped me deal with my past and process it. Trauma affected my self-esteem. He led me through that until I became more confident and could talk about what had happened and tackle the world again. I had time to heal, build myself back up, and find myself.

He started to help me recognise my self-worth, set boundaries, and realise what's good and acceptable and what's not. When your confidence is in your shoes, you accept bad behaviour. It's like you feel you deserve poor treatment. That was how I lived for a long time. I'm still learning, even now. I've come to understand that while you can have strong self-worth, some people will mistake kindness for weakness and try to exploit it. But that's not because you lack self-worth – it's because they have little integrity and are pursuing their own agenda. Never let undeserving people undo your healing progress.

In the end, I kept going. And I guess I thought of those managers and became even more determined. I'll show you. Nobody will ever speak to me like that again, and no one will bring me down like that again.

I have become a far different person from the one I was when I first met Paul and Aisling in 2018. The one aspect of my life I didn't expose to therapy was my eating disorder. I had never been diagnosed, but I knew. I never discussed that with Paul. I kept that part of me under wraps, and that turned out to be a mistake because it soon came back to bite me.

23

In Training

After the inquest, Mam and I felt despondent. We were convinced that if we didn't learn more about what had triggered Alan Hawe's killing spree, more innocent families might be murdered.

Then the words of an eminent psychologist gave me renewed hope for pursuing a proper inquiry. Days after the inquest, the head of St Patrick's mental hospital wrote a newspaper article saying depression shouldn't be used as the first excuse in murder-suicides.

Dr Paul Gilligan said to blame mental illness for Alan Hawe's deeds without any level of certainty was deeply stigmatising. 'Those with mental-health difficulties are no more likely to commit violent crime than others and ... are more likely to harm themselves,' he wrote.

The CEO of St Patrick's health services also posed an important question: 'Did Alan Hawe murder Clodagh and Liam, Niall and Ryan because he had mental-health difficulties or because he was angry and distressed?'

I was relieved. At last, I thought, a professional who does not automatically associate murder-suicides with depression and mental illness. The association of the two seems so insulting to people with mental-health problems. People with depression don't go around killing their entire families. There had to have been something more at work.

Shortly after reading his article, I heard Dr Gilligan speak on the radio. He came across as someone compassionate, down-to-earth and approachable. I thought he might be able to point us in a new direction because, by early 2019, Mam and I felt at a dead end. But what would this doctor think about a random call from a stranger asking him for help?

By then, we had been told the investigation into Clodagh and the boys' murders was over, and the case was closed. There had been no progression in the case since the inquest, or if there was, we weren't told about it.

The investigators were guarded about telling us anything. Their reluctance to pursue the case boiled down to one fact – Alan Hawe was dead. What did it matter? There was no one to convict, no criminal trial to prosecute. The inquest had decided he murdered everyone after a bout of long-standing depression. So, what was the point in investigating further or giving us more information?

Our meeting with the investigation team in Cavan garda station on 17 January 2019 was a disaster. It was clear that they were only concerned with a potential data-protection breach or accusing me of approaching a witness.

'I would like you to leave with the assurance that every avenue was looked at and we got every answer,' the lead detective said. But if they got every answer, they didn't share it with us, the victims' family. They seemed determined to keep us in the dark and hope that, eventually, we might go away.

After that meeting, we approached our solicitor and asked him to request the gardaí file for the investigation. We weren't too surprised when we received a letter in return, refusing our request. The gardaí cited data protection and confidentiality.

'Where do we go now? What next?' I asked Mam. I knew we'd reached the end of the road with this investigation team. Clodagh and the boys' file had been locked away in Cavan garda station, destined to gather dust.

All four lives were reduced to murder statistics and a reference number, which was how the investigation team intended to keep it. Somehow, we needed to reopen the investigation or get a new one under way, but I had no idea how.

During our January meeting Mam told the gardaí in Cavan that we would go public with our story. But we sounded more defiant than we felt. We didn't have a clue how to go about doing that properly. We needed the backing of the wider public if we were going to get anywhere. And we needed to make a lot of noise to be heard.

The last thing I wanted to do was go public and speak about the murders and the investigation. But I also knew Clodagh and her boys would be forgotten unless we did something, and I couldn't let their deaths be in vain. I was now determined there would be some meaning to what had happened to them – that they would leave an important legacy.

After reading Dr Gilligan's words in a newspaper and hearing him speak on the radio, I felt he was on the same wavelength. We had been trying to broadcast the same message. We didn't believe depression was the root cause of the murders. Alan Hawe was not depressed. Nor was he a psychotic man who had suffered years of mental torment and then exploded or 'snapped'.

The way he had carried out the murders of his wife and children was as premeditated and cold as a professional assassination would have been. Claiming that Alan Hawe was mentally ill and not responsible for his actions felt like a cop-out, an easy means of explaining away something that was far more sinister and calculated.

Clodagh and her children's murders are, unfortunately, only one of a succession of murder-suicides in Ireland. Our case is far from the only familicide in the country, but it has the unfortunate distinction of being the largest. The former state pathologist, Marie Cassidy, first raised concerns about the large numbers of family 'annihilations' she saw in Ireland not long after she arrived here from Scotland in 2004. Mam and I felt obligated to do as much as we could to minimise the chance of it happening again.

After working in hospitals in the past, I knew Dr Gilligan would have access to a communications department. I wondered if he might be sympathetic to our cause or if he or his team could point me in the direction of how we could go public and bring attention to our case. I was apprehensive, but I dialled the office number for Dr Gilligan anyway.

I told his office who I was, explained that Dr Gilligan had written an article that referred to our family and asked whether I could speak to him. I had no idea how he would feel about someone cold-calling like this. While I was doing my shopping in Lidl later, he returned my call.

Mam and I arranged to meet Paul at the hospital within days. He listened and engaged with us and said he would try to help. From that day on, he took us under his wing. We were blessed. Thanks to him and Tamara Nolan, director of communications at the hospital, everything started to snowball.

Paul was astute enough to realise that if we wanted to go public and spread our message, we would need professional help. 'As you have no experience with the media, I think it will help if you have training,' he said. 'And I know just the person.'

That was how Mam and I were introduced to the former Dragons' Den TV star, media consultant and entrepreneur Gavin Duffy. He agreed to train us to face the media. We first met him in St Patrick's hospital, and then we started training with him at his house, Kilsharvan, on his country estate near Bellewstown in County Meath.

'What are the important messages?' he asked. 'Let's focus on the points you want to make.'

We wanted the public to see Clodagh and the boys as the real flesh-and-blood people they were, not crime statistics or murder victims. We wanted to explain how we owed it to Clodagh and the boys to seek the full truth about why Alan Hawe murdered his family that night.

We were determined to call for changes to the Succession Act 1965. We wanted the government to change the law so that a spouse murderer or child killer could not benefit financially from their victim's death.

But most of all, we said we wanted access to the garda files of the investigation and a new, more thorough inquiry into our family members' deaths.

We sat with Gavin Duffy for weeks, and he looked after us with tea, biscuits and first-class training. He'd say things such as 'Jacqueline, stop throwing petrol bombs. You can't say something like that. We can talk about this subject, but not like that.' I just laughed, but then he'd show me how to say what had to be said without causing legal headaches for ourselves or the media.

Gavin was such a kind and gentle man. What Mam and I learnt during our time with him was invaluable. We honed our message and gained enough confidence to come out and face the cameras for the first time in our lives. All we could do now was hope that by speaking out we could unlock a dusty filing cabinet in Cavan garda station and start pursuing real justice for Clodagh and the boys.

24

Going Public

The first time Mam and I met with RTÉ's current-affairs presenter Claire Byrne, I wasn't sure what kind of person to expect. Dr Paul Gilligan had arranged everything. He rang Jane Murphy, who was then a producer with *Claire Byrne Live*, and it all happened very quickly after that.

First we met with both women in St Patrick's hospital. The idea was to discuss the possibility of an interview on *Claire Byrne Live* where we would talk about the case for the first time, reveal our unhappiness with the investigation and call for a new inquiry into our family's deaths.

Claire listened more than talked at that first meeting. Off television I had expected her demeanour to be professional, analytical and methodical. But her TV persona belies the warmth and emotional maturity of the person we met and came to know. She had a quiet presence and showed a spirit of humility and empathy that I hadn't expected. Moreover, as a wife, a sister, a daughter and a mother, she empathised with everything we were feeling. She and Jane made a great team, both kind and generous with their time. It felt good, even refreshing, to deal with other women for a change.

They never put us under pressure, making us feel at ease with them from the start. 'This meeting doesn't mean you have to do this interview with me,' I remember Claire saying. 'Take your time and consider your options.' We had offers from other programmes and media outlets, but we trusted Claire and Jane from the first time we met. They understood the trauma we had experienced and were receptive to what we wanted to achieve from appearing on the programme. They worked hard to provide a calm, safe environment to talk.

We learnt that Clodagh and the boys' story would be aired on national television as a *Claire Byrne Live Special*. Live TV seemed too much pressure, though, so it was agreed that we would pre-record our interview. In no time, it was all organised. I knew we had the perfect platform to campaign for a new investigation, and now it was up to us to get our message across clearly.

After that initial meeting with Claire and Jane, we continued our media training. I remember spending the evening of my thirty-eighth birthday in media training with Gavin, thinking, *Isn't this just great?* Not that Gavin isn't a lovely person, but having constantly to repeat myself, rehearse and memorise facts was not my idea of a celebration.

Claire kept in touch and let us know we could pick up the phone to her or Jane at any stage if we had any concerns. Our interview was scheduled to be recorded on Friday, 22 February 2019, just a month after we had met with the garda investigation team in Cavan.

Gavin had schooled us well. We knew what we wanted to say and the questions we needed answered. I felt we were in safe hands with Claire and Jane. But I was still petrified as I arrived at RTÉ, and we were led down a warren of corridors to a dressing room. Appearing on national TV on a current-affairs programme was way out of my comfort zone. So much was riding on it for us, and there was no plan B. This was our last chance to appeal for a proper investigation, to get real answers in Clodagh and the boys' case and we wanted to get it right.

We had watched RTÉ all our lives but had never dreamed we would find ourselves at the station and part of a programme focusing on our family. It felt surreal to be there, behind the scenes. By the time they came for us and led us to the studio for the recording, I was sick with nerves.

The studio was fitted out like a sitting room with couches and side lamps. It looked so cosy and intimate that some people asked afterwards whether the interview was filmed in my house or Mam's. I remember the heat from the lights, and

I hoped no one could see me shaking as the cameras were trained on us and Claire began with her questions.

We told our stories as best we could, considering how nervous we were. We described Clodagh, Liam, Niall and Ryan, then concentrated on raising our questions and concerns about the murder investigation. I felt edgy and tense throughout, but anytime the stress or upset got too much, we were able to stop. We had someone looking after us all the time, and we could go outside for a walk to clear our heads.

The *Late Late Show* band was rehearsing for that night, and Claire's production team had to stop and start our recording as their music could be heard in our studio. I had the novelty of walking down to the *Late Late Show* studio and peering in to see what was happening. I met Ryan Tubridy and got a photo with him. Derek O'Connor from the Camembert Quartet showed us so much kindness. We spent countless hours recording the interview; Claire, Jane, and the entire production team gave us the time and space to discuss the tragedy in depth.

We finally left RTÉ that Friday night at around 9.30 p.m., mentally and physically exhausted. I was seeing double as I drove home to Cavan, but I also felt heartened. We had spoken out for the first time, poured out so much of what we wanted to say, and the people on the show had taken the time to listen and record it all.

'What do you think, Mam? How did we do?' I asked, on the way home.

'We've done our best, Jacqueline. We can't do any more.'

Still, as I returned to RTÉ the Monday after, anxiety gnawed at my insides again. We were to view the entire interview at 2.30 p.m. before it aired as *Her Name Is Clodagh – A Claire Byrne Live Special* at 9.35 p.m. that night.

Jane played the recording for us, and I watched with a sick feeling – anxious about our performance and apprehensive about the reaction to the programme. Parts of the interview made my heart sink, and I thought, *Oh, God, I could have said that better.* I cringed to hear and see myself, but I suppose no one likes looking at themselves on television.

Mostly I was worried about the public reaction when it aired that night. Would we get any support? Would there be any reaction? Or would people say, 'Look at this pair, only dying to get their faces on the television'? If only they knew how much hard work, sleeplessness, stress and anxiety were poured into that one interview. I had no idea what to think or how the programme would be received.

After the screening, we returned to our hotel in Ballsbridge with Carmel and Gerry, Melissa and Eileen. They continued to support us in our efforts to get a second investigation into the murders.

We returned to the RTÉ studio for the broadcast of our interview and the live segment of the show that night. The audience was tiny: our family members, Gavin Duffy and his wife Orlaith, and the Social Democrats councillor

Gary Gannon, who had started the social-media campaign #HerNameIsClodagh. He sat next to me that night, with Mam on my other side.

The knot in my stomach tightened as I watched our interview being screened to the nation. Then Claire hosted a live panel discussion with guests who included Kathleen Chada, whose two boys, Eoghan, aged ten, and Ruairí, five, were murdered by their father, Sanjeev Chada. Also on the panel was Margaret Martin from Women's Aid and forensic criminologist Dr Monckton Smith from the UK.

Dr Monckton Smith said similar domestic homicide cases and experiences had been seen in the UK, the United States, Canada and Australia. She also said greater awareness needed to be shared with the wider community and police to prevent or predict these murders.

'Unfortunately, this case reflects my experience of many cases like this,' Dr Monckton Smith said. 'We like to think that this is something that doesn't happen very often. Unfortunately, that isn't the case. These behaviours are known about.'

Claire hammered home our message during the panel discussion. 'The very least the family deserve is a full picture of how it came to this point on that night in August of 2016,' she said. 'And they don't have that tonight, and they're begging for all that information.'

'Of course, they want that information,' replied Dr Monckton Smith. 'But we all want it as well ... How are we going to learn? How are we going to stop things like this happening in the future?'

It felt like a triumph to hear experts confirm what we had been trying to say all along. But I was still worried sick about how the programme would be received. Would it pass unnoticed? Would people be critical of us going public? Would people be like the authorities and say, 'Let this go. They're all dead. The file is closed. Forget about it'?

The signature tune marking the end of *Claire Byrne Live* played, and then everything started. The response to the programme was almost immediate. #HerNameIsClodagh began to trend in the minutes after the show, and my phone blew up with an outpouring of support. It was beyond belief. I couldn't keep up with the texts and messages from Facebook, Twitter and WhatsApp.

'Mam, you've got to see this!' I said. I was stunned as message after message poured in. Social media exploded with support and expressions of anger at our treatment. I exhaled, really exhaled, for the first time in months. The reaction was fantastic. We'd needed to know we had done right by putting our faces into the public arena and speaking out. We badly needed that validation, and we got it. That night, we felt a massive wave of support from the general public and sensed that the tide was turning.

'Maybe we'll get the answers now, Mam,' I said. And my heart lifted for the first time in months, and I started to hope again.

25

The Phone Call

When Mam and I got home the following afternoon, we headed for the graves at Castlerahan. I needed quiet reflection after all the stress of the previous days.

The newspaper headlines had been full of Clodagh and the boys that morning after *Claire Byrne Live*. Some newspapers even published the entire transcript of our interview. Radio stations nationwide discussed the case, and the public was angry to hear how our legal system had turned its back on our family. The full glare of the media spotlight was on our story, along with our request for a new and more thorough investigation into the murders.

When I need to think I like to retreat to the graveyard. The solid permanence of the old church and the solitude of the leafy surroundings are always calming. I spent time that afternoon tending Richie's grave, updating him on Gary's progress and sharing the latest news about the campaign for Clodagh.

I left Richie's grave and joined Mam in the shadow of St Mary's Church, where Clodagh and the boys' grave is located. The internal dialogue continued. *What do you think, Clodagh? Can you believe the reaction we got from being on television last night? I think we did the right thing, but what do you think our next step should be?* I didn't know how to exploit all the media attention to our advantage.

My phone's urgent ringtone shattered the serenity of the cemetery. It was a Dublin number, one I didn't recognise, but I answered the call anyway.

'Hello. I'm Charlie Flanagan, the minister for justice,' the caller said. 'Is this a good time to talk?' To have the ear of the justice minister seemed like the answer to our prayers after a three-year struggle.

When politicians began reacting to the programme, I gave a wry smile. Nobody from the state sent their condolences or attended the funeral when Clodagh and the boys were murdered. A family of four was murdered, and there wasn't a sound from a politician. A week afterwards, the children's minister, Katherine Zappone, was quoted at an event saying the murders saddened her, but that was it.

Following our interview with Claire Byrne, politicians tripped over each other in the Dáil talking about their sadness, the need for action, and changing laws. I was cynical. I knew a lot of the response was lip service and playing to the public gallery, but at the same time, I was grateful that our story was on the political radar at last.

Fianna Fáil leader Micheál Martin spoke in the Dáil about our courage and loss and added: 'There are many disturbing elements to this story, and many of their questions have remained unanswered for far too long ... The family wants basic answers.'

Sinn Féin leader Mary Lou McDonald said anyone who saw the programme was deeply affected. 'It is clear from the testimony of Clodagh's family last night that they need answers. The state also needs answers. As legislators, there is an onus on us to ensure the necessary statutory provisions are in place to understand in full how and why these violent crimes occur,' she added.

Mary Lou said she had written to Garda Commissioner Drew Harris and the justice minister asking to introduce domestic-homicide reviews. 'Organisations such as Women's Aid have long advocated the introduction of such reviews in this country,' she said. 'The family and friends of victims should also be included in the review process.'

I was particularly heartened by Taoiseach Leo Varadkar's contribution to the Dáil that day. I had written to him before and never received a reply. He spoke about our case and also referred to the Monageer family murder, in which twenty-four-year-old Ciara Dunne and her two daughters, Lean, aged five, and Shania, aged three, were found murdered at their home in Wexford in April 2007. Ciara's twenty-nine-year-old husband, Adrian, was found hanged after strangling and suffocating his wife and daughters. In this case, there were red flags. He had enquired in advance about the cost of coffins and a funeral for the family. Despite this, they all died.

The taoiseach said the Department of Health regarded 'familicide' as a criminal issue for the Department of Justice, but both departments needed to coordinate on such matters. Awareness-raising programmes on coercive control were already happening in garda divisions around the country.

More importantly for us, he added: 'The minister for justice will be very happy to receive a submission from the family with their suggestions, and perhaps we will take it from there.'

That was the cue for Charlie Flanagan to call us in the graveyard. My conversation with the minister was friendly and brief. He sympathised with us on our losses and commended us on our interview the night before. Then he invited Mam and me to attend a meeting at Government Buildings that week. He said his office would be back in touch with the arrangements.

I got off the phone, relieved. So, it had worked. We had achieved what we wanted by baring our souls on *Claire Byrne Live*. It was sad that we had needed to go to that extreme. Mam looked at me enquiringly. 'It's happening, Mam. We have a meeting with the justice minister this week.'

After that it all came together very quickly. The *Claire Byrne Live* programme was broadcast on Monday, 25 February 2019, and by Thursday afternoon, we found ourselves being escorted through the doors of Government Buildings.

We felt prepared. Before the meeting, we had had another session with Gavin Duffy. He also coached us on how to address the media afterwards. He warned us again to be 'on message': 'This is what you say. This is what you ask for. And don't elaborate.'

Gavin had been a vital cog in the success of our campaign so far, and we didn't want to mess up this next step so we were grateful for his input again. Even after our coaching session, though, walking into Government Buildings was intimidating. The prospect of a meeting with the minister for justice was another experience way out of my comfort zone.

I was a bundle of nerves going in, even though Tamara Nolan, St Patrick's hospital's communications director (and, by now, a personal friend), accompanied us. Part of me was already fretting about being interviewed by the media afterwards. I worried I might say the wrong thing and bring the whole house of cards down on us.

I didn't need to worry about the now former minister Charlie Flanagan. As soon as we were escorted to his offices, he bounded out to welcome us and took my extended hand in both of his. He insisted on making tea in his private office, and when I went to help, he whipped the teacups off me. 'Don't you dare!' he said. 'I'll make your tea. You sit down and put your feet up. I make the tea around here!'

Two officials, both women from the Department of Justice, also sat in on the meeting, and everyone did their best to make us feel at home. We presented Mr Flanagan with a prepared list of ten requests, helping to keep us and the meeting on track.

We asked him to release details of any investigation conducted by the school into Alan Hawe. We told him about Hawe's conflict with a work colleague, his contact with the INTO, and his words that the truth was going to come out. We asked the minister to assist us in getting information from the Department of Education, Tusla or the coroner who conducted the inquest.

We called for reviews into the homicides of women and children to learn from them and prevent further tragedies. We also discussed reforms to Irish inheritance law and legislation to block the relatives of people like Alan Hawe, who kill family members, from profiting from murder.

But as a matter of priority, we asked Mr Flanagan to allow us to review the garda files and launch a new investigation into the murders of Clodagh and the boys.

I was expecting defensiveness, which seemed to be the knee-jerk attitude of everyone in authority we had met so far, but Charlie Flanagan disarmed us with his humanity. He was kind, warm and normal. We had a ninety-minute meeting with him, and we left with the assurance that he would arrange a meeting with Garda Commissioner Drew Harris. He was more than happy to address our other issues too. I felt a lot lighter leaving that meeting than I had in a long time. Finally, someone in authority had listened to us and even understood and agreed with us on many of the subjects we raised.

'We're feeling very positive that changes will come from this,' I told the media afterwards. And I did feel positive. Two and a half years after my sister and nephews were murdered, it seemed we were finally making progress.

26

Social Media

In the aftermath of *Claire Byrne Live*, I was scrolling through Facebook one night when I stopped, blinking in shock. A graphic at the end of the post caught my attention first. The headline was white on a large red square background and read: #Istandwithcastlerahanns. My heart started pounding. *I stand with Castlerahan national school.*

I read the lengthy post and reread it, struggling to comprehend why someone would write that. The post, several hundred words long, wounded me to the point I was physically sick. I remember gripping the bathroom basin, trembling violently, sobbing so hard I couldn't catch my breath.

I had been astonished by the outpouring of support in our town of Virginia after our RTÉ appearance. Walking down the street shortly after the programme aired, a complete stranger stopped me. 'I had no idea what you were going through,' she said.

People I hardly knew started pulling me in for hugs. The entire community of Virginia seemed to wrap their arms around us, which surprised me because we were new to the town, blow-ins. Yet when we sat in the local hotel, we were told our order was on the house. People approached or sat down with us, and 'We had no idea' was a common theme. How could they have? We were so quiet for so long. We were silenced out of fear a lot of the time. I was always afraid I'd jeopardise the investigation or the inquest by speaking out, so I didn't.

I still wasn't comfortable in the media, but we'd decided to expose ourselves to its spotlight. After being trained, I felt some confidence. Facing the press wasn't as traumatic as it had been during the funerals and the inquest. I still found the exposure difficult at times.

A Sunday newspaper invited me to write an article about the investigation afterwards, and Gavin organised a photographer. I scrolled through some of the comments online when it was published, and my stomach lurched when I got to the one that read: 'She looks very well for someone who's supposed to be grieving.' Despite mostly positive comments, that one hurt. I read other stinging remarks on social media, usually callous or silly, about how I looked or what I wore, and each wounded me.

I still felt that going public was worth any abuse. Clodagh and the boys had a chance of getting justice at last, and if I could help stop someone else going through the pain I still endured, speaking out was worth it.

But the #Istandwithcastlerahanns post was the most hurtful thing I have ever seen on social media. Mam and I spoke about our difficulties in the wake of the murders on *Claire Byrne Live*. Despite everything that Alan Hawe wrote in his murder letter – that he was caught red-handed and dreaded going back to school – we said we had never found out what was going on in his work life. We were still in the dark.

I stated that we had never spoken to anyone from his school since Clodagh and the boys died. Nobody had approached us to give us the information we needed.

After the programme aired, we heard RTÉ had received letters of complaint from people living in Castlerahan. I raised my eyes to heaven. Some locals felt a murder-suicide was not good for the image of the area. They believed by talking about it, we were tarnishing the reputation of the place and all those living in it.

I thought it was the reaction of a handful of people. But I hadn't expected to read the type of hostility expressed in #Istandwithcastlerahanns. The author opened by referring to the 'tragic story of the Hawe family' and continued by praising the teachers and 'the beautiful country school that is Castlerahan NS'.

The post continued: 'I commended the teachers and staff for making it so in spite of the tremendous horror that they have had to endure' and referred to 'people and a community being ripped to shreds over this horrific tragedy. They should be commended for what they have done against horrific and unnatural odds, and not condemned over hearsay.'

The poster called on readers to 'fight fire with fire and show our support for Castlerahan NS on social media'. Without ever referring to us, the poster attacked our family and accused us of casually castigating the school and the community of Castlerahan.

Did these people know that four people had been murdered? Did they realise that some people in the school had failed to provide statements to the investigation into the murders? How would they feel if this happened in their family? How did they expect us to react? We just wanted the answers to which we were entitled.

I knew the advice. I could almost hear my psychologist Dr Paul Gaffney telling me to back away from negative social media, but I couldn't help myself. I knew I should switch it off, but I didn't. I read and reread the post and the comments after it. I flinched seeing comments from people Clodagh had thought were friends. I read comments from people I recognised – including business owners in Virginia. Many people shared the post – some I knew. I was awake until 4 a.m., rereading it, ruminating, crying, getting sick.

My sister and nephews were integral to the community of Castlerahan. Of all places, I thought the people there would be our biggest supporters. I still struggled to understand how some people in that school refused to help the investigation even though four people were murdered, including two of their pupils – two young boys. Yet, the only sympathy in that Facebook post was for the pain and inconvenience the school had had to endure.

I wanted to reply to the post, but I couldn't. I badly wanted to defend ourselves, but I knew the media would pick it up, and any public skirmish would only distract from what we ultimately wanted to achieve.

I remember screen-grabbing the post and sending it to Jane Murphy in RTÉ. Claire Byrne rang me and scolded me. 'Put the phone down. Don't be looking at your phone!' Of course she was right, but I couldn't help myself. I found it so upsetting. That morning, everyone else in the family read it. We were all distraught.

Thankfully, the post was taken down a long time later, but it still hurts that it was ever put out there. The most hurtful thing of all was that throughout that entire post there was no mention of Clodagh, Liam, Niall or Ryan. Throughout the hundreds of words in it and the many comments afterwards, not a single person mentioned the four victims, members of the Castlerahan community, lying in their graves right across the road from that school.

27

The Commissioner

On Thursday, 7 March 2019, a week after meeting Charlie Flanagan at Government Buildings, Mam and I arrived at Garda Headquarters in the Phoenix Park in Dublin. We were brought through security and escorted into the grand Georgian building.

We were there to meet with Drew Harris, the former deputy chief constable of the Police Service of Northern Ireland, who was only months in his new job. He had set about creating an improved policing culture and was the new broom sweeping clean the organisation.

There was much talk about the old boys' club being disbanded and a new modern way of policing being heralded. We hoped to find a man who would be open to reviewing the investigation into the murders and see the necessity for launching a new one. However, our welcome from the new garda commissioner was cooler than the one we received from the minister for justice.

We were brought to what appeared to be more of an elegant dining room than a meeting room. Elaborate drapes framed the windows, gilt-framed oil paintings hung on the walls, and an ornate table stretched through the centre of the grand room.

Mam and I sat with Tamara Nolan and Gavin Duffy on one side of the table. The commissioner, the assistant commissioner for the north-western region, Barry O'Brien, and another senior garda faced us. I was not naive enough to expect an effusive welcome at Garda Headquarters. I was well aware that the meeting would never have taken place had it not been for the furore sparked by *Claire Byrne Live* and the intervention of the minister for justice.

But the moment the senior garda officers sat opposite us, I sensed the familiar polite-but-frosty atmosphere from previous meetings with the guards. Mr Harris was an icicle in the room, his bearing rigid and his demeanour remote. It became clear that in the days since our meeting with the minister for justice, he had talked at length to the lead detective on the investigation in Cavan. From the start of the meeting, he sounded like the same detective repeatedly trotting out the same interminable phrases: Every avenue has been investigated … can't force people to make statements … can give you our assurances that …

Oh, my God, I thought. *This is going to be the same as our meeting in Cavan garda station in January.*

Despite the high ceilings in the room, I felt the air pressing down on me. My despair only grew as the meeting progressed. We were facing another brick wall. I remember thinking, *He doesn't give a shit what we're saying to him. He's not listening. He's just running down the clock.*

Gavin Duffy spoke out several times. I'd love to have the minutes of that meeting to relate what was said. Several times, I've requested them from the guards and others, and they're not forthcoming. But I was glad to have a male presence on our side of the table. I often find men are less dismissive of the opinions of other men. I felt that the gardaí were not budging. *Sure, you know everything. Didn't the investigation team tell you everything they learnt?*

'We don't even know the time of Alan Hawe's death,' I said. 'We asked the investigation team on numerous occasions, and we were told they didn't know. If we don't even know that, how could you say we know everything?'

Mam and I continued to argue. 'What about the missing envelope in the school, the one Alan Hawe saw with his name on it?' (The guards said they only found a file containing his CV.)

'What about the witness who reported seeing Alan Hawe out and about hours after he was supposed to be dead?'

'Why wasn't there a luminous forensic test for blood done on his car?'

'What did Alan Hawe ring the INTO about?'

'Who caught him "red handed" and why was it about to "blow up" in the school?'

'When you're still left with these questions after a woman and three children have been murdered, how can you just go and close the file?' I asked.

We fought our corner as the minutes ticked on, but the main man on the other side of the table was unyielding, and I grew increasingly upset. I was crying. Mam was crying. Tears of frustration and fear. After all we'd been through, Drew Harris was going to refuse our request for a thorough investigation.

The meeting was nearing its conclusion. We had said all we had to say and were getting nowhere. Reason, argument and logic were not working. Appealing on the grounds of justice and humanity was not working. I felt desperate. We had come this far, exposed ourselves on national television and met the minister for justice. I couldn't leave that room without the promise of an investigation. *What is going to work here?* I thought desperately.

Instinct and personal experience kicked in. Not many like to be in the eye of a media storm, and I imagined the garda commissioner wouldn't want to be in a whirlwind of controversy during his honeymoon phase in his new job. I also knew public sentiment was on our side since our interview on *Claire Byrne Live*.

'Well, there's a lot of media waiting outside,' I said. 'What do you want us to tell them?' He suggested the guards leave the room for recess.

We waited. I had a flicker of hope now but still had no idea what the outcome would be. When the gardaí returned to the room, Drew Harris suddenly announced they had agreed to sanction a case review from the serious crime review team under the assistant garda commissioner in the room. We looked at each other, unsure of what that meant.

'That means there'll be a new investigation?' I ventured.

'Pretty much,' said Drew Harris.

After a long battle, we'd got exactly what we wanted, so you'd imagine we might have cheered or high-fived each other in jubilation. But after a lengthy and emotional few hours in Garda Headquarters, the case review was hard-won. We were punch drunk and drained from stress, frustration and tears, so there was no sense of celebration. There was only relief.

We were still dazed when we met with the media outside to reveal that An Garda Síochána had agreed to establish a review into the murder of Clodagh and her three children.

We also said we had been inundated with messages since the RTÉ programme and were grateful for the support we received from everyone. And we meant it. The authorities had tried to silence us and nearly succeeded, but they couldn't silence the public outcry and the media.

28

Succession

I haven't been back to Clodagh's house since the funerals. Neither has Mam. The red-brick dormer, which Clodagh had made so homely and cosy, has lain dark and empty, the curtains still drawn since that night. I don't even travel down that road any more.

Photos of the house were published a couple of years ago. They appeared with a touching remembrance of Clodagh and her boys, written by the *Anglo-Celt*'s Seamus Enright. I was shocked, seeing the garden, once manicured and mown, looking so wild and overgrown. The family cars lay abandoned, and Alan Hawe's silver Kia Sportage was covered with creepy streaks of algae slime. Clodagh's once lovely family home looked so desolate and grim. My heart sank seeing the devastation.

I wanted nothing to do with the house for a long time. Mam and I never wanted it, and we tried not even to think about Clodagh's home, now lying empty. When these matters finally reached probate, we were told that the house had value and would sell. Selling was something I'd never even considered. 'Who'd want to live there?' I asked, horrified at the thought.

We were told, People forget. Someone from outside the area, probably Dublin, would buy it. It was heartbreaking to hear anyone could forget what had happened in that house. Instinctively, I didn't want another family in there. It would be awful to think of another woman and children living where Clodagh and her children had once lived. It felt wrong.

Such evil happened there that night that I don't feel it would be a safe place for any family. I'm a spiritual person, and I believe the energy in that house could not be good for anyone after four lives were taken in it.

Mam and I soon realised that we wanted the house because we didn't want it sold to anyone else. Even though we decided to fight for it, we still didn't know what we wanted to do with it. We only knew that neither of us wanted the house to be sold. However, from early on, we realised we had no control of Clodagh's house or any of her estate because, by law, everything was now in the hands of the murderer's family.

As soon as Alan Hawe murdered our family, he had inherited everything that belonged to them, according to an outdated and archaic law, the Succession Act 1965. And when he killed himself, his next of kin, his parents, had inherited everything from him.

For a long time after the murders, probate and succession rights didn't matter to us. Clodagh's estate and belongings didn't enter our heads. We spent nine months pursuing Alan Hawe's exhumation and waited sixteen for the inquest. Probate couldn't even begin until after the inquest and we received a verdict of unlawful killings.

And when the issue of probate was raised, it was never about money for us. It was the principle of not allowing Alan Hawe to control everything even after death. But we knew that we had a battle on our hands to ensure that the Hawes didn't inherit Clodagh's money as well as everything else.

Once we decided we wanted to fight for the house, it weighed heavily on our minds. What were we going to do with it?

In the ensuing battle with the Hawes, we had three priorities: to make sure Clodagh's estate did not go to the murderer's family, to get control of the house, and have the funeral costs paid.

Soon after the inquest, we had everything ready to go. Our solicitor, Liam Keane, put us in the hands of one of his colleagues, Anjana Hanratty, an expert on probate. Nothing happened in the entire year following the inquest, and there was nothing we could do because everything was in the Hawes' control.

Our only saving grace was the legal clause or precedent set in the Celine Cawley case, a woman killed by her husband, Eamonn Lillis, in Howth, County Dublin in 2008. Eamonn Lillis was convicted of manslaughter by a jury in 2010, and a lengthy battle ensued between him and Celine Cawley's family over property jointly owned by the couple.

By law, Lillis was entitled to inherit everything they owned jointly. The case came before the High Court, where the survivorship rule was modified to prevent him from acquiring Celine Cawley's share of their property. The High Court called for legislation on the matter in 2011, but nothing had happened to make it law.

Mam and I went to the Four Courts in January 2019, hoping that, through mediation, we could get a legal agreement on the same grounds as the Celine Cawley case. It would mean that Clodagh's share of the property would not automatically go to the Hawes. It was a horrendously stressful time. The two legal sides sat in separate mediation rooms in the Four Courts, toing and froing between each other. We declared all of Clodagh's sole and joint assets, pension, life insurance policies, salary protection, credit union money, et cetera.

But it was a massive waste of time, stress and effort. The legal team for the Hawes declared only €20,000 in assets for Alan Hawe. Meanwhile, the cost of meeting the barrister twice and hiring her for one day's mediation well exceeded that amount.

We already faced debts of €50,000 in inquest legal fees and funeral costs, and the bills continued to pile up. Mounting debts were a constant worry, especially for my mother, who was retired and on a pension. It was just one battle after another. We tried not to worry about the costs – justice was the important thing. But it seems people need wealth to afford justice in this country. We didn't realise that this was just the beginning of the legal bills in the process. (By the time probate was concluded, eight years after the murders, we had built up legal costs of €180,000.)

Stephen Hawe was appointed administrator of Alan Hawe's estate at the end of February 2019 for the purpose of defending legal proceedings against the estate. His wife, Olive, immediately started personal-injury proceedings against her son's estate, which included a claim for damages for trauma due to the murders.

In April 2019, we initiated personal-injury and nervous-shock claims against Stephen Hawe in his capacity as the legal representative of Alan Hawe's estate. It was a strategy to ensure we had some kind of claim on Clodagh's estate. That started a protracted legal dispute with the Hawes over the proceeds of Clodagh and Alan Hawe's estate.

The Hawes were legally entitled to everything Clodagh owned. However, they gave a guarantee to accept the ruling in the Celine Cawley case, which meant they wouldn't claim Clodagh's assets. If they hadn't accepted the Celine Cawley case ruling, Section 120, we would have had to incur huge costs going to the High Court.

We also requested that Alan Hawe's estate pay for all the five funerals he had caused. The undertaker waited five years to be paid until the Hawes released their son's money to pay for the funerals in 2021. Our personal-injury and nervous-shock claims also had to come out of Alan Hawe's estate, which meant we got the house in the end.

We succeeded in getting Clodagh's estate, thanks to the efforts of Celine Cawley's relatives, who got that High Court ruling to stop Eamonn Lillis from profiting from his crime. But that High Court case was in 2011, and all these years later, that court ruling is still not legislated for.

We have seen new bills being brought forward for stalking and coercive control, and there have been dozens of other changes in the laws in this country. Yet lip service is all we've had concerning succession laws and domestic homicide. Mam and I were dragged through years of hell with legal wrangling, solicitors, mediation and courts because the murderer's family was in control.

We called on former justice minister Charlie Flanagan to reform Irish inheritance law. He duly pledged to initiate changes to block those who kill family and relatives from profiting from the crime.

Fianna Fáil TD Jim O'Callaghan tried relentlessly to push legislation through. Sinn Féin and Mary Lou McDonald's office wanted to push through legislation. Justice Minister Helen McEntee said she would push through a new bill.

So many politicians spoke about the necessity for this legislation after our interview with Claire Byrne, but it's been talk and no action. What is the resistance to this change? Why are we still waiting for a bill to close this loophole in inheritance law allowing a spouse or their successors to benefit financially from domestic homicide?

Any new legislation will make no difference for us. Probate was finally settled in December 2021 and only concluded in April 2024. But if the law is changed now, it will make a difference to other families. Domestic homicide and murder-suicides are not as rare as they might once have been.

The issue of the house continued to weigh on our minds. Mam and I still didn't want it, and we knew we wouldn't sell it. We started asking ourselves what Clodagh would like us to do. I visited a faith healer in Monaghan a couple of years ago and spoke with him about it. He suggested Clodagh would like the house demolished and four oak trees planted in its place in memory of her and the boys. It was as if a weight was lifted off me as soon as he said it.

Mam thought about it and agreed that Clodagh would have liked that. And that was it. I've already been in touch with Cavan County Council, even though the probate agreement hasn't been fully signed yet. They said it would cost €50,000 at that time to demolish the house, take it away and landscape the plot. It was a shock to discover that the cost of something so fundamental, not just to us as a family but in the interest of the community as a whole, would need to be borne by the victims and not by the county council. But this was the reality we faced into.

After Mam and I submitted the planning permission to demolish the house, I saw critical comments on Facebook. One person branded it as wasteful to demolish a valuable house. I felt no urge to respond to someone who had no clue. The building is no longer a home or a house: it's a murder scene.

The discussion became whether we should demolish it with the contents or not. Neither of us wanted to go back in there, and I didn't want strangers going through the place. I already had a box of their possessions but I can't bear to open it, and the thought of walking through the house again made me feel physically sick.

Of course Gerry, the family hero, stepped forward once again. He has volunteered to clear the house with the help of a handful of close friends. We will be forever grateful to Gerry, Carmel and their girls for their unwavering love and support. We're a small family but very close.

The house and its history of horror will be razed to the ground. Mam and I are determined no one will ever be able to buy the site or build on it. We will plant four oak trees and place a plaque and maybe a bench there as a peaceful place in Clodagh, Liam, Niall and Ryan's memory. The site will hopefully remain a little garden of remembrance for Clodagh and the boys for ever, a small haven of peace and tranquillity in their memory.

29

Serious Crime Review

The question was one of hundreds posed by the detective that day in the overheated garda station, but it hit me like ice water in my face. 'Do you know that Alan Hawe saw you as a threat?'

I was speechless for an instant. I knew Alan Hawe constantly tried to demean me. He was smug and self-assured. But I never once guessed that he regarded me as a threat.

As I grappled with that possibility, the detective lobbed another grenade. 'Do you know every text message you ever sent to Clodagh was forwarded to Alan Hawe?'

My mind paused, struggling to absorb those words and the magnitude of their meaning. Then, I felt a surge of anger. I remember thinking, *Jesus, Clodagh, why the hell would you do that?* Fortunately, this information emerged near the end of my interview with the serious crime review team because Clodagh forwarding my texts was all I could think about afterwards.

By then, I'd spent the entire day in the victims' interview suite at Stradone garda station in Cavan. These suites are purpose-built spaces in a few places around the country. Each looks like a modern, comfortable office environment rather than a typical garda interview room. However, after nine hours of answering questions, the relaxing surroundings did little for me. I felt drained.

The review had got under way almost straight after Mam and I met with Drew Harris in March 2019. Assistant Commissioner Barry O'Brien came to my house soon after. I first met him at the meeting with Commissioner Drew Harris but didn't gain any real insight into him in Garda Headquarters. However, I distinctly remember Barry walking into my house a week later because he stopped to admire a photo collage of Gary's first year. Straight away, I recognised a family man. He retired in 2022 before the serious crime review team completed their report.

The assistant commissioner introduced me to the head of the team, Detective Superintendent Desmond McTiernan, whom I fondly referred to as 'Super Des'.

Based in Harcourt Street in Dublin, the team, often called the cold case unit, tries to identify new leads in major unresolved cases. Its motto is 'To the living, we owe respect; to the dead, we owe the truth' and, from the start, we received respect and communication from everyone we dealt with. It was like night and day between the two investigations.

I soon discovered they were all family people. Des and his right-hand man, Brian Quirke, who was then a detective sergeant, are tall, burly men who are always dressed immaculately in suits. They're shrewd professionals, and yet they're warm human beings, who have compassion and treat everyone around them with dignity.

Most of our dealings were with Des, the head of the team. From the beginning, he was completely invested in finding out what had happened. With Des, I could ring, text, be in touch and get a reply. There were no 'them and us' boundaries as we had encountered with the original investigators. 'This might be a stupid question—' I said once, but Des cut across me. 'No question is stupid, Jacqueline. You ask me whatever you want.'

Above all, the investigators on this team related to Mam and me and empathised with us. Des called me the first time he entered Clodagh's house the following month, April 2019, and I heard the catch in his voice. He was affected by being in a place where a woman and three children were murdered. He could understand what it would be like if it had happened to his family. From the day they started on the case, we felt that we were listened to and heard.

The team went to the ends of the earth in their work. They investigated every little detail. I suggested they talk to the couple who owned SuperValu in the town because they coached Niall's basketball team. They did and found more information about the night of the murders than we had ever expected.

The initial investigators played down Hawe's use of adult material, only telling Mam and me that it 'wasn't porn as we know it'. The review team uncovered the depth of his obsession. Within months, we were learning that what they discovered was extremely dark in nature.

Mam and I had been told we would be the last witnesses interviewed as part of the review. We were finally called in September 2021. Mam went in first, and I was brought in the day after. The victims' interview suites in Stradone are equipped with the best audio and video recording equipment. Des was in the recording room with another detective, while Brian Quirke and a colleague were in the interview room with me. Both helped to make the day as easy as possible.

Trauma is a thief. Post-traumatic stress disorder doesn't just take away your sense of safety and trust but can also impair your memory. I don't recall a lot of what went on during those nine hours, but I remember they asked many questions beginning with 'Did you know?' or 'Do you know what this means?' Sometimes, they showed me a photo or suggested a name and most of the time, I replied that I didn't know the answer. I remember they listed endless pornography and live sex sites they'd found on Alan Hawe's devices that I'd never heard of.

Near the end of the interview, one of the detectives read a brief definition of coercive control: 'Coercive control is a persistent pattern of controlling, coercive and threatening behaviour. It includes all or some forms of domestic abuse (emotional, physical, financial, sexual, including threats) by a partner or ex-partner. It traps women in a relationship and makes it impossible or dangerous to leave ...'

When Clodagh was alive, I'd never heard of coercive control, and I certainly wouldn't have identified the signs. Sitting in the garda station that day, I was painfully aware of what it meant and how I had failed to recognise it in Clodagh's life.

I only grasped the extent of Hawe's psychological and emotional control over Clodagh after discovering she had forwarded all my phone texts to him. She was in an abusive intimate relationship in which she was monitored and manipulated.

I've no idea what covert tactics and mind games he used to make her forward my messages. But I understand now that she couldn't see clearly because of his hold on her.

I don't even know if Clodagh ever realised she was in an abusive relationship. As an abuser, he disguised himself well. Clodagh was an intelligent woman, yet he was able somehow to distort her thinking and her life to suit himself. He no doubt presented his version of life as the ideal family dynamic.

At first, I still couldn't help feeling angry about what

she had done. Whatever her relationship with her husband, Clodagh and I were sisters. Sisters have a different relationship from husband and wife, so it felt as if she had broken my trust and betrayed me. I continued to feel like that for a while, but now I know what control and manipulation look like. It wasn't Clodagh's fault, and she was probably appeasing Hawe. A person in love or deeply invested in a relationship often experiences a gradual shift in their reality. It's much like the frog in the boiling water story. The water is so slowly warming that the changes are imperceptible to the frog. Love and trust create blind spots, and concerning behaviours are rationalised as care or protection. I've experienced it myself. When someone you trust offers explanations for your nagging doubts or concerns, it can feel easier to accept their version of reality than to confront the red flags or consider the possibility that they're manipulating you.

The mind is remarkably adaptable, and where manipulation is subtle, even a highly intelligent person can unconsciously adjust their perceptions of reality to maintain the relationship, particularly when the perpetrator plays on deep-seated hopes or insecurities.

I rarely emailed Clodagh as I knew she and Alan shared an address, and he read everything I sent her. But never in a million years did I suspect she was forwarding all my text messages to him.

I asked the detectives, but they couldn't see why or when

this arrangement was made. She forwarded everything apart from a couple of photos she had deleted rather than pass them on to her husband.

I still can't read back over those messages. I can't change anything, and it would be just too painful in so many ways. I'm not angry with Clodagh any more. I understand why she did what she did, and I prefer to think about the times when I needed her, and she was always there. She was there for me when Richie died and when Gary was born.

Alan Hawe and I tolerated each other for appearances' sake, but he never wasted any opportunity to point out how irresponsible and silly I was. He made me feel as if the way I was living my life was wrong, chiefly because I like to socialise and enjoy myself.

The serious crime review showed me that he saw me as a threat because he couldn't control me. He knew I didn't admire or respect him and feared I might learn too much or influence Clodagh somehow. He made sure to drive a wedge between us. He monitored all my communications with Clodagh and tried to keep me at a distance in case I might reorient her thinking. I just wish I'd realised all this sooner.

I also wish I had known that Clodagh was beginning to disengage from him and was seriously thinking of ending their relationship. But I would never have guessed she was doing this because I firmly believed they had the perfect marriage until the day she died.

The review report landed on Drew Harris's desk in 2023. He was not prepared to release it or provide us with a copy but finally allowed the team to brief us on the findings. And so, five years after the review was set up, on a cold morning on 12 January 2024, the senior investigators gathered in my mother's kitchen in Virginia to present their findings.

Detective Superintendent Des McTiernan led the presentation as head of the team. He was joined by former Detective Sergeant Brian Quirke, who had since been promoted to inspector and national interview advisor with the Garda National Bureau of Criminal Investigation. Also present was Detective Garda Michelle Wallace.

They set up a PowerPoint presentation with forty-five slides on a screen. Des said the report was eight hundred pages long, with another three hundred of appendices and other references. He explained it had been a challenge to contain four years of work into a presentation format.

A marathon ten-hour presentation followed as Mam and I sat rigid in the kitchen, listening to the three detectives. I tried to absorb the cascade of information coming at me, interjecting with questions when I didn't understand.

Brian did all the talking while Des sometimes interjected, adding extra details. Brian told us that the second investigation team faced a challenging scenario when entering Clodagh's home for the first time in April 2019.

Of the original 122 exhibits collected in the 2016 investigation, nearly half had been destroyed. The original investigation could not be criticised for this as they were compliant with standard policy and procedures. But I could never understand why the family's bloodied clothing was destroyed while an Aldi brochure from the coffee-table was kept. I was glad it was retained, however. Through careful analysis of indentations they found on it, the team discovered that Hawe's murder note had been written in the sitting room. He had sat on the couch, hunched over the coffee-table, writing page after page, sitting beside my murdered sister. When he had finished, he placed his letter in the kitchen. It was a chilling detail that helped piece together a far fuller picture of the murderer's callous and calculating actions that night.

Despite the setback of fifty-six destroyed exhibits, the review team generated 226 new exhibits that were overlooked by the original inquiry. They assembled the physical evidence with methodical precision. They returned to the house four times and found a secret Wi-Fi phone and many other items the original investigators had missed.

Dr Stephen Clifford from Forensic Science Ireland was called upon to analyse blood splatter. Once Hawe had cut their throats, the expert determined, none of the victims had moved significantly. Distinct areas of bloodstaining surrounded Clodagh, each telling its own part of the story. Blood spatter in front of the couch was found on a holiday brochure, an Aldi brochure, and Clodagh's phone and mug. A pool of blood on the floor beside the knife and hatchet was caused by Clodagh's position on the couch or from the weapons. The original blood samples in the house were no longer visible, except on Niall and Liam's beds. We requested information regarding who had died first, but a ballistics team and Dr Clifford couldn't make any definitive statement based on the evidence remaining.

The now-retired state pathologist, Dr Michael Curtis, who had conducted the original post-mortem examinations, stated at the inquest that Hawe killed Clodagh before killing Liam, Niall and Ryan in that order. This sequence seems to be the most likely order of the killings.

The review team looked into Hawe's visit to SuperValu Xtra-Vision on the last day anyone saw them alive. He rented two movies, *Gone Girl* and *The Purge*. The team examined their rental history and saw that the films were not representative of their usual family-friendly ones.

Inspector Brian Quirke had the foresight to take the DVD player back to their Dublin offices. (The electricity had been cut off years earlier.) Once he plugged it in, out popped Hawe's copy of *Gone Girl*. I reeled as the team outlined how both movies contained themes that eerily parallelled the coming violence.

Gone Girl opens with a monologue from its star Ben Affleck (playing Nick Dunne), stating, 'When I think of my wife, I always think of her head. I picture cracking her lovely skull, unspooling her brain, trying to get answers.' The words were so sinister in light of what he planned to do. The same movie also features a pivotal scene in which a character's throat is cut.

The Purge is a dark and dystopian movie about a night when crime (including murder) becomes legal in America. It also contains a scene in which a character's throat is cut. The film focuses on the chaos and violence during the 'purge' night. Hawe's forethought and planning were disturbing. He deliberately picked these movies for some twisted reason, maybe to psych himself up for murder.

The digital evidence uncovered in the house painted another disturbing picture and revealed more of Hawe's scheming. The team found he used four different cache-cleaning apps. He wasn't merely clearing storage space: the number of apps suggested a deliberate pattern of concealment.

Hawe and Clodagh shared an email address, Alan& Clodagh@. However, the team also found that Hawe had created a secret John Smithers@ email account in September 2004 to access porn sites. Twelve years later, when Clodagh died, I'm sure she still knew nothing about it.

They also found and examined a secret SIM-only phone, which the initial team failed to see. The mobile worked on Wi-Fi only, which meant no bills were associated with the phone, and Clodagh would have been unaware of it. Investigations revealed it was used to access pornography. Hawe may have feared Clodagh could check his laptop and his official mobile, so he stashed this other phone. Detectives couldn't link the mobile directly to Alan Hawe, but on the balance of probabilities, they believed it was his.

According to their report, it contained traces of hundreds of pornographic images, some of which were classified as illegal content. They found more than four hundred images already wiped from the phone. Thirty-six images that were recovered were classified as concerning, and ten were confirmed as illegal child pornography. He had an image with the gay dating app Grindr on it. They cannot say if he ever used the service. He might have googled it, but it was deleted through the cache so the team couldn't retrieve further information. Also on the phone were videos of elderly people having sex.

The team were very open with us, saying that Hawe had had serious sexual issues. 'He didn't know what he was,' was how one of the team assessed him. Unfortunately, they couldn't access emails on his 'John Smithers' account as the data was held in America.

The investigation also requested data from Instagram for two accounts. Their request was again rejected in America. The European headquarters of Meta (formerly Facebook) cooperated after Inspector Brian Quirke got a warrant. Meta's European management flew over from London to give the team the data they needed.

Hawe's bloodstained hands used Liam's phone at 12.08 a.m., 12.10 a.m., and 12.39 a.m. on Monday, 29 August, which confirmed the family were dead by then.

The software team from Meta confirmed the activity on the phone, but they couldn't determine why Hawe had used Liam's phone that morning due to the considerable lapse in time. Hours later, at 3.08 a.m., Hawe made his final bank transaction, stopping payments for the car insurance due the following day and the next mortgage payment of €2,500. That digital footprint helped establish the timing and the calculating nature of what he did.

The investigation also looked into other strange calls Hawe made before the murders. After an online pornography search on 28 January 2016, Hawe made a six-minute call at 2.30 a.m. He made a second call even later that night to the same number. The review team tried to investigate the nature and the reason for the calls. They discovered the person whom Hawe called was a recovering porn addict, so detectives said he and Hawe shared an addiction in common. When the investigation contacted him, the man would not cooperate. He accused the team of fabricating the calls, then said he couldn't recall them. Ultimately, he failed to account for what was discussed during the calls, and the team had no power to arrest someone who didn't provide information. Why were two porn addicts on a phone call in the middle of the night? What were they discussing? Why or how did they meet? It was bizarre. All we know for sure is that Hawe had a secret life that Clodagh and the rest of us knew nothing about.

Clodagh's phone revealed a different story. The review team

confirmed that Google searches between December 2015 and August 2016 painted a picture of a woman contemplating significant life changes. She had looked up articles that indicated she was considering separating. Contrary to the original investigation, which said she looked up 'parenting alone at Christmas' in December 2015, she was reading this mere hours before she was murdered. Her search history strongly indicated that Clodagh was considering leaving her marriage. Their shared email address meant that Hawe could (and probably did) monitor her searches.

Digital searches showed Hawe had researched several murder-suicide cases. He looked up a case in 2014 involving Valerie Greaney (forty-nine), who was fatally stabbed by her husband, Michael Greaney (fifty-three), at their home in Cobh, County Cork. Before killing himself, Greaney also stabbed their daughter Michelle, who survived. Hawe looked at this article several times on 22 August, days before he committed the murders. They also found articles he had used to research murder-suicides and stabbings a year earlier.

Their findings helped establish timelines, behaviour patterns, and details that were overlooked in the original investigation. While some of our questions remained unanswered – locked in encrypted files or deleted histories – the digital trail provided new insights into the night's events. They pointed to a calculated sequence and uncovered details crucial to understanding the murders.

The investigation dispelled any notion that Hawe's actions were spontaneous.

Hawe's laptop also contained links and searches for dating and porn websites. He accessed a site called Covenant Eyes that markets itself as a tool for users to stop engaging with online pornography. The team went through legal channels in the US to see if he had subscribed, but the site wouldn't engage.

The review team were also able to refute Hawe's claim in his murder letter that porn pop-ups would appear on his laptop because he used ClipConverter. They confirmed that visiting the website alone would never create a pop-up.

The investigation team's findings on Clodagh and Alan Hawe's cars proved inconclusive. While no blood was found in either the Renault or the Kia, retired pathologist Dr Michael Curtis confirmed Hawe could have driven without leaving blood traces. His bloodied clothes and the cuts on his hands from the murders would have dried by late morning.

The man who had approached me and said he'd seen Alan Hawe that morning was re-interviewed. Upon investigation, they discovered he had been in hospital that morning, so it wasn't physically possible for him to have seen Hawe at Burrough Hill as he had claimed. Instead, the team found a new witness who claimed he had seen Alan Hawe at Burrough Hill on the morning of 29 August. They used enhanced cognitive interviewing and memory techniques to bring the person back in time. The review team went to great lengths to investigate his claim and verify his testimony, checking appointment times and travel durations. They found everything supported the witness's account of seeing Hawe that morning.

They tried to follow up the sighting with CCTV evidence, but critical footage that might have answered questions about Hawe's movements had either been lost or was never gathered.

The handling of the CCTV evidence was particularly concerning. The review team found that footage from surveillance cameras had never been collected or viewed. Gardaí from Virginia had claimed to have canvassed three specific houses near a crucial junction, but when the review team followed up, householders confirmed these visits had not occurred. This CCTV footage can never be retrieved.

The second investigation team checked the angle of one camera and believed it would have been ideally placed to capture footage of Alan Hawe if he was, as we suspected, going to the school that morning.

Castlerahan school had no proper alarm system. Everyone used the same code to enter, and the keypad had no memory. Brian checked Hawe's keys and confirmed he could have accessed the school at any time. After their investigations, the review team concluded, on the balance of probability, that Alan Hawe was on the road that morning and heading towards the school.

This meticulous gathering and analysis of evidence

contrasted starkly with the first investigation. They high-lighted how much the original investigation had missed. The serious crime review team provided crucial answers to many of our questions. Some mysteries – such as Hawe's exact movements that morning – remain unsolved because the first investigation failed to collect and preserve CCTV evidence.

Paul Collins, a forensic engineer, conducted experiments regarding the ligature used by Hawe to kill himself. His work with rope stretching and weight tests helped establish a more precise timing of events. He believed Hawe died sometime around 7.30 a.m., many hours after he had murdered everyone else.

The team re-examined 115 witness statements taken during the first investigation. They found that witnesses were interviewed without the expertise needed and that statements lacked critical detail.

Brian Quirke is a highly skilled garda interviewer. His team identified thirty-six witnesses who needed re-interviewing, twenty with advanced techniques. They also interviewed 286 additional witnesses during the second investigation. According to the report, the original investigation should have used detectives with level-four interview skills. Those more skilled detectives should also have conducted enhanced cognitive interviews with the witnesses. The original murder investigation failed to request this available expertise.

Hawe's counsellor was a significant witness. Despite being mentioned twice in the murder letters, he gave only a prepared statement eight months after the murders. Gardaí had no opportunity to ask follow-up questions. The review team were also critical of the guards for not interviewing the counsellor immediately after the murders.

Brian interviewed the counsellor and asked about his scant notes from his sessions with Hawe. He also queried why he had never asked his patient more in-depth questions. The counsellor maintained that his role had been 'to listen, not judge'.

Many questions remain unanswered. So much time had elapsed that many details of the counselling sessions are lost for ever. If advanced interviewers had been used in the first investigation, they might have gathered more information.

I have other questions I'd like answered. I realise counsellors have an ethical obligation to maintain client confidentiality. However, there are exceptions when there's a risk to the client or others. Could an assistant school principal's succumbing to sexual urges in a school be regarded as risky behaviour and warrant intervention? Do counsellors have a duty to report a potential risk to minors? The detective asked the counsellor at which school and where Hawe had been masturbating. Hawe had never told him. The detectives believe that it was most likely Castlerahan national school.

The team cleared up issues concerning the school laptop, which was said by the first investigation to contain pornographic material. The review team discovered the first investigation soon realised the porn had come from an inadvertent data transfer – a detail they failed to communicate to us or anyone. This misinformation left a cloud of suspicion on what had happened at the school that should never have existed. The guards' failure to address questions and communicate with everyone involved caused a lot of distress to us and others.

The review team found lists of school staff among Hawe's belongings, which led to new lines of enquiry. Nine witnesses from Castlerahan national school were re-interviewed. This time, the interviews were recorded rather than simply written down, ensuring that no detail, no matter how small, would be lost.

The review team's approach was thorough. They interviewed Castlerahan's teachers, special-needs assistants and members of the management board. Still, some declined to participate – four refused outright while another couldn't engage for medical reasons.

The review team confirmed the 'toilet' incident when Ryan was ordered to clean up a wet floor. The incident was never mentioned in board of management meeting minutes. We learnt that Clodagh and Hawe wrote to the school, both signing the letter, complaining about Ryan being told to clean the floor. We were also told that Hawe was asked to leave the room during a staff meeting on 15 June when the issue was discussed with the teacher involved.

The serious crime review team interviewed the school's

principal in October 2019. Hawe had told Clodagh that the principal ran out of the school and went straight to Father Kelly's house. However, the principal said she felt intimidated and bullied by Hawe on 21 June 2016 during a meeting to clear the air. But she said she spoke only to her husband about the incident and never made any official complaint about Hawe's behaviour. She said no investigation of Hawe was pending.

The review team also tried to interview Father Kelly before he died. They spoke to his doctor in Cavan general, who advised that the priest wasn't well enough to be interviewed. After he died, the team reviewed Father Kelly's original statement, which stated that anything Alan Hawe discussed with him was confidential or confessional privilege. He also said in his statement that he didn't understand what had happened. Investigators regarded Father Kelly's statement as ambiguous. The team pursued alternative avenues, interviewing those who knew him. They discovered that Kelly had attended a counsellor, whom they also interviewed. The counsellor said the priest didn't disclose any information concerning Hawe.

Staff in Castlerahan and other schools said they had had no concerns about Hawe, and nobody had filed grievances against him. They had found no specific proof that he had been masturbating or looking at porn at the school, apart from his admission to the counsellor. This behaviour was likely conducted on his personal laptop and in the men's toilets. No one witnessed it. They uncovered nothing more about the file that Hawe was so concerned about. They confirmed it contained only his CV. We will never know if he got to the school that morning to remove something else.

The review team confirmed that Alan Hawe had called the Irish National Teachers' Organisation (INTO) three times. They believe these calls were only general enquiries. They found no complaints or anything concerning. They found no evidence of Hawe's claims that he was 'caught red-handed' anywhere. They found no answers to why he 'dreaded going back to school' and what he meant by the 'truth would come out'.

A witness at the inquest described 'a clump' of hair found in the house, probably Clodagh's. The picture that the description evoked always bothered Mam and me. However, the second investigation team said the description was inaccurate and offered to show us a photo. Mam left the room, but I looked at it: it was a few strands of hair and did not resemble 'a clump'. It's not right for anybody to have to spend years after an inquest seeking answers because of a word that was said in the courtroom, which led to more questions than answers.

The review team also spent months exploring whether Hawe suffered from a psychosis linked to Hashimoto's thyroiditis. The team was passed from one medical practitioner to another, looking for insight into the disorder.

They consulted experts from specialist labs in the UK, France and Germany. Ireland's chief state pathologist, Dr Linda Mulligan, was helpful and practical in the matter, according to the report.

Theories about sudden psychosis were carefully examined and dismissed. Dr Michael Curtis, who had conducted the original post-mortem examinations, said the thyroid condition was coincidental.

He found no evidence of bipolar or of Hawe experiencing a psychotic episode. Dr Curtis's evidence, combined with analysis from state laboratories, helped establish that there was no physical basis for claims that Hashimoto's thyroiditis, psychosis or other medical conditions could explain Hawe's actions.

The review team revealed that Professor Harry Kennedy, a key expert hired by the state for the inquest, declined to engage with the second investigation. I was astonished. He had explained Hawe's actions as the result of severe mental illness and claimed Hawe had suffered from depression for years.

His conclusions were among the reasons Mam and I requested a new inquest into the murders of our family. Our solicitor asked for a meeting with the attorney general to discuss it. We also discovered there was neither an audio recording nor a written transcript of the inquest proceedings, with no stenographer present.

Without further input from Professor Kennedy, the

review team had to look for new experts to help with their investigation. Scottish forensic criminologist Professor David Wilson prepared an enlightening report for the team instead.

He identified key characteristics of what he termed a 'family annihilator' – a classification with recognised behaviour patterns. Hawe's killings match the research that says Sundays are the most common day for such murders to be committed. Professor Wilson noted research shows that the incidents are becoming more common and are less likely to be explained by mental-health issues.

Instead, his report says familicides are linked to control, and that family annihilation is often planned by men masked as loving fathers and husbands, who harbour deep-seated fears about their masculinity and social standing. The professor noted that such individuals plan their actions carefully, and their outward appearance of normality covers internal turmoil.

His report also noted 'pseudo-altruistic' comments in Hawe's murder letter. Hawe's statements might have appeared caring but reflected a desire to control how events would be interpreted after he had killed his entire family. He wanted people to see his murders as an act of mercy or protection, a way to spare the family from future suffering or disgrace.

He perceived Hawe's murder letter as an attempt to control and manipulate. He believed it was a selfish attempt to temper the readers' judgement, and his suicide was a move to avoid the criminal justice system.

Professor Wilson pointed out elements of narcissism, saying Hawe saw the family as extensions of himself. He believed Clodagh and the boys were possessions to do with as he pleased, a common theme among family annihilators. Hawe's actions were about power and control, and prompted by fears of 'social death'.

The concept of 'social death' is another common theme in family annihilation. The perpetrator's perception is that he is losing control, including the loss of his social identity. Hawe became preoccupied with perceived threats to his status and feared things were about to 'blow up'. His role in the school provided income, structure in his life and status in the community. He feared losing his status as a husband and father and losing authority and respect within the school. For Hawe, that amounted to 'social death'.

Professor Wilson believed it significant that Hawe killed everyone the day before returning to school. The school was another location for masturbation. He also noted Hawe's cross-dressing and erectile dysfunction issues, which dated back to 2012; he had been prescribed Viagra by his GP. Hawe's perceived disintegration of his body and inability to perform as a man added to his fears of social death. He believed he catastrophised everything and said it was impossible to identify the tipping point.

Professor David Wilson took no payment for his work in

the investigation. I am very grateful to him for his insight into what might have precipitated Clodagh and her boys' murders.

The expertise of Professor Ella Arensman proved valuable too. For more than thirty years, Dutch-born Professor Arensman had conducted research into suicide, self-harm and public mental health. She has studied the nature of murder-suicides, noting that Ireland had seen a shocking fifty-one such cases up to 2020.

She believes that murder-suicides should be considered a major public-health issue. In her report, the professor said the effects of these crimes ripple through communities long after the immediate tragedy. She also believes murder-suicides are linked with personality disorders such as narcissism.

According to the professor, Hawe's letter showed disconnection, a need for control and a distorted reality. She, too, believed that he regarded Clodagh and the boys as possessions. She also noted his 'altruistic' comments in his murder letters. She said Hawe's behaviour was typical of many murder-suicides in some ways. However, his systematic actions and detailed instructions were not common among other murder-suicides she had investigated.

She thinks Hawe could have masked a major depressive disorder for up to twelve weeks before the murders, despite evidence that he was researching stabbings a year before he killed everyone. She also refuted suggestions of coercive control in his behaviour. I'm not sure how she would otherwise describe his monitoring of Clodagh's and my communications. The professor's report was extensive, and I am only scratching the surface here because I don't have a copy.

During the review team's presentation, they clarified that Clodagh had mistakenly forwarded one text back to me instead of to Hawe. She explained it to me as 'a dizzy moment'. They said she continued to forward all my messages to her husband.

The experts' combined analysis painted a picture of planning rather than impulsivity, and control rather than chaos. They highlighted that Hawe's actions aligned with known patterns of family annihilators – especially his attempt to control the narrative after death.

The serious crime review team concluded that the murders were planned. Hawe's sexual-based fears and problems were central themes, as were significant personality-disorder traits, including obsessive-compulsive characteristics. Through interviews with colleagues and family members, a picture emerged of someone who demonstrated rigid perfectionism and a preoccupation with order and control. Mam recalled that Hawe rearranged Ryan's pictures and magnets in the playroom into orderly lines only shortly before killing him.

The report claimed that Hawe exhibited excessive concern around rules and morality. He struggled with change and catastrophised minor events into major crises.

We learnt that the Hawe family was surprised to receive a phone call from him on 28 August because he had only recently visited. The investigators didn't say what time they received this call. In hindsight, the Hawes realised he was saying goodbye. A colleague contacted Hawe by text on 22 August, and Hawe replied, saying, 'Mass exodus next Monday.' The colleague didn't understand what he meant by that. The report confirmed that Hawe had lost contact with any friends. He was a loner, isolated apart from family, and had no friends.

The review laid bare significant shortcomings in the original investigation, which fell below the required professional standards. What was initially treated as straightforward has proven far more complex. The team identified three major areas where the original investigation had failed.

First, they identified the mishandling of CCTV evidence. Two gardaí were referred for disciplinary procedures regarding CCTV failures. We were told that, after an investigation, a decision would be made about the alleged misconduct. If the guards were found guilty of breaching discipline, various sanctions might be applied, ranging from a warning or reprimand to more severe penalties, such as suspension or dismissal. The process was handled internally, so we don't know who the guards were, and we won't know the outcome unless they appeal the decision of the disciplinary procedure.

Second, the report stated the original murder investigation

team conducted superficial computer and phone data analysis. It was also critical of the original investigating team for missing crucial digital evidence.

Third, the review team was critical of witness interviews, where key testimonies were collected without proper expertise.

The report also called for fundamental changes in procedures for preserving evidence. New guidelines were proposed to extend retention periods for exhibits, particularly in cases involving murder-suicide. In our case, phones and clothing were destroyed before the second investigation opened.

The report emphasised that murder-suicides should receive a thorough investigation like any other murder, regardless of the perpetrator's death. The original garda team deemed the mass murder of a woman and her children as a coroner's investigation. They didn't apply any of the rigour of a criminal investigation.

The serious crime review team have recommended that in future, they treat such cases as though they were proceeding to the director of public prosecutions, ensuring the highest investigative standards.

They also recommended improved crime-scene logging procedures and enhanced witness interview protocols. The team proposed that level-four-trained interviewers should be made available nationally.

They advocated structural changes, including supervisory

checks for similar cases and higher professional standards for murder-suicide investigations. They recommended the appointment of an incident-room coordinator for these crimes.

The review team emphasised the need for a victim-centred approach in all investigations. They acknowledged that while the original investigation had provided a service, it had failed to deliver the professional standard that victims' families deserve. Brian apologised to Mam and me for the first investigation team's failings.

They said the recommendations had already begun influencing garda training at Templemore. Senior officers were now being taught to approach murder-suicides with the same rigour as any other homicide. This has given me hope that the report will be a watershed moment, prompting a fundamental shift in how such tragedies are to be investigated in future.

By the time the presentation was over, daylight had tracked around the house and faded to darkness. The review team's thoroughness had been both a comfort and a torment. I felt comforted that they had gone to the ends of the earth to find out what had happened, but hearing some of the revelations was torture.

My mind felt as if it was brimming to overflow at times, unable to contain one more detail. It was ridiculous that we had to hear the entire report in a single presentation rather than receive it to read in our own time. But I understood this was the decision of those much higher up the food chain than the serious crime review team.

I want to express my heartfelt gratitude to them all. Their head, Detective Superintendent Des McTiernan, takes justified pride in his people, and they are a testament to his leadership. He is a consummate professional and a gentleman. I will never forget speaking to Des the day he first stepped into Clodagh's house. His reaction was so humane, and I could hear how the experience impacted him, even on the phone. He treated Mam and me like his own family. Des has a gentle soul and always showed genuine concern for our ordeal. His empathy shines through in everything he does.

He also communicated continuously throughout the process. The subject was sombre, but we always found something to laugh about. I'm relieved the process is largely behind me, but I miss our chats.

I also want to extend my deepest thanks to Brian Quirke, interview advisor, Garda National Bureau of Criminal Investigation, another true gentleman. His professionalism is unmatched in my experience, and the country would be a better place if every garda shared his work ethic and principles. If he were to become our garda commissioner, he would bring much improvement to the organisation.

I listened to the report presentation over those ten hours to try to understand the full scope of what had happened. The second investigation team explored every avenue and bottomed out every lead. They brought us closure on many issues and revealed more about the cold, twisted and manipulative stranger married to Clodagh. By the end of the presentation, I realised greater knowledge might not bring peace, but it had at least ended some of the uncertainty.

With the help of the serious crime review team's report, I understood Alan Hawe felt Clodagh slipping from his control. At first, he tried to regain her trust by making a show of pained guilt and going to a counsellor. But he lied to her, to the counsellor, to the GP, to everyone. Hawe had no intention of changing his behaviour, only appearing to do so. Clodagh could never have known that threatening Alan Hawe with separation was a high-risk strategy. She never realised that the quiet, oppressive force in her home was also deadly.

I think back to Dr Paul Gilligan's question in his article: 'Did Alan Hawe murder Clodagh and Liam, Niall and Ryan because he had mental-health difficulties or because he was angry?' From the start, he was perceptive enough to understand why Hawe murdered everyone.

Alan Hawe believed something in the school was about to 'blow up'. He also felt he was losing control at work. For whatever reason, he thought his mask of respectability and his privileged position in the community was about to slip, and he knew that when Clodagh found out she would definitely leave him.

But his hubris wouldn't allow him to face the consequences of his actions, and the mere thought that Clodagh would even consider leaving enraged him. He couldn't countenance the humiliation of being disgraced in his community, and his outraged sense of entitlement couldn't bear to let Clodagh or the children enjoy their lives without him. He saw Clodagh, Liam, Niall and Ryan as his possessions, pawns to do with as he chose. With his back to the wall, he moved to his endgame.

We have always suspected there was a trigger to Hawe's actions, and I still believe someone out there may know the truth. However, I must accept that we'll likely never know what it is. All we've ever wanted is the truth of what happened that summer.

It's nearly nine years since Clodagh, Liam, Niall and Ryan were murdered in a crime that shocked the country. Clodagh should be forty-eight this year, still working as a teacher. If she had lived, I'd like to think she would have left Hawe and would be happily living her best life, maybe in a second relationship. She would be looking on proudly as her eldest, Liam, now twenty-three, would be close to graduating from college. Niall would be a young man of twenty this year, maybe pursuing his dream of becoming a baker or a chef. Little Ryan would be fifteen, still at school, and sitting his Junior Cert. Instead, all that potential and life is gone, and they're lying in St Mary's churchyard in Castlerahan.

Mam and I participated in an independent study examining best practices in conducting domestic-homicide reviews in Ireland. The study was commissioned by the Department of Justice and published in 2023 as the 'Study on Familicide and Domestic Homicide Reviews'. As part of the family consultation group, we urged for policy changes in inquests that attract media attention. We emphasised the importance of appointing coroners outside the county to ensure impartiality. We also highlighted the enormous financial implications for families: our legal fees after eight years amounted to €180,000.

Mam and I have also asked the minister for justice and the garda commissioner to publish the findings of the serious crime review team. The report was finalised in 2023 and gathers dust on a shelf somewhere in Garda Headquarters. We're told that they will not publish the report for operational reasons. We've heard they may have fears that publicising the details of the murders might risk copycat crimes.

However, I believe it's vitally important that they are not kept under wraps. Women, men and children could benefit from the findings, which include expert analysis of a family annihilation case in Ireland. Potentially, they could lead to improved policies and better accountability within An Garda Síochána. Policymakers, non-governmental organisations and other stakeholders could also glean valuable information and provide more effective strategies for the prevention of and intervention in murder-suicides.

The report is the culmination of a four-year comprehensive investigation, and taxpayers' money was used to compile it. Let's break the silence and learn from the insights it provides.

Mam and I owed it to Clodagh, Liam, Niall and Ryan to find out as much as we could about why they died. Thanks to the serious crime review team report, we've come a long way. The next step is a second inquest into my sister and my nephews' deaths. A new and better-informed inquest could also help highlight issues and recommendations that may help prevent similar deaths in the future, we hope, negate the original findings of Professor Harry Kennedy.

The report revealed that more than fifty cases of murder-suicide were identified in the years up to 2020. So many women and children have been innocent victims of these crimes. The thought of other women and children needlessly dying underscores the urgency of our task to push for release of the report and hold a second inquest. Anything we can do to stop such grief and destruction happening to another Irish family should be done. I know it's what Clodagh, Liam, Niall and Ryan would have wanted.

30

Healing

Healing from grief is often overwhelming, and wounds of lost love can run so deep that raising your head from the pillow feels impossible some days. I'm not an expert on healing, but I've learnt that while the pain may not disappear, it slowly makes room for hope and light.

The process of grieving for Clodagh, Liam, Niall and Ryan has been complicated by the ongoing struggle for truth and justice and the stress of settling their estate. Even now, with legal matters resolved, the brutal nature of their deaths weighs heavily on me.

Few people, thankfully, can comprehend the pain of loss from murderous violence. On my own stumbling journey, I've learnt that time doesn't heal these wounds. Rather it teaches us how to live with them. With suicide, which also leaves unimaginable pain in its wake, acceptance comes slowly too. You learn to cope and accept it more as time goes on. You move forward, but the grief remains.

As you grieve, you must also navigate a new life path in your other relationships, whether with family, friends or romantic interests. One of the hardest lessons I've learnt is that people often judge those who have experienced trauma. They may withdraw or perceive us differently, driven by discomfort or fear.

Following the murders of my sister and nephews, I expected people to be sympathetic and understanding, considering the trauma thrust upon our family. Instead, I discovered that, like mental-health issues, trauma carries its own stigma, often creating a second wound. Survivors not only have to cope with their loss but also with being treated as somehow 'other'.

Many friendships I once had have dissolved since the murders, as some people have recoiled from my family's profound tragedy. I understand that they can't bear to confront the raw reality of tragedy striking so close. They can't fathom how such senseless violence could touch someone they know. It shatters their careful illusion that horror happens to strangers in distant places.

Sometimes people also seem to have an irrational fear that tragedy might somehow be contagious. They withdraw from a painful situation to protect their own sense of safety.

Others may retreat because they feel helpless in the face of such devastating loss. What words could possibly matter? Rather than risk saying the wrong thing, they say nothing at all. They convince themselves that the grieving family needs space and that their presence might be an intrusion until their distance becomes a habit.

However, those who, deep down, need to believe that terrible things happen for a reason cause most pain: they can't accept that bad things happen to good people for no reason. Grieving people become stigmatised and isolated because some want to avoid any social association with those 'tainted' by trauma.

Anyone like me, who has experienced such profound losses, is likely to develop PTSD. The nervous system becomes severely compromised, and certain triggers are inevitable, yet there is a lack of understanding and education about the effects of trauma. When I've shared these triggers with trusted individuals, I've expected them to be understood and respected. Instead, people have said and done things that have triggered and even deepened my grief and trauma. I've had people question my mental stability and make comments to friends like 'How could she be right in the head?' or 'That's not normal behaviour.'

Some remarks have been made in ignorance, but others have been cruel in their intention. Either way, I've had to develop greater resilience against them.

Clodagh's words always come to mind: 'We shouldn't

be defined by what happens to us.' This came after she experienced others' judgement after losing our brother Tadhg. The pattern sadly continues. People should remember that great loss doesn't make a person unstable: it simply means their heart has been shattered. Yet many people have tried to reduce me to my past experiences.

None of the traumatic events in my life were of my doing. I wasn't related to Alan Hawe, and my husband's actions were the result of his own hidden pain. Yet I discovered that matters little in some relationships, especially romantic ones. In more recent years, as Gary got older, I've embarked on a few and regretted a couple.

Some years ago, I was in a brief relationship with a man who commented over dinner that I had eaten my whole calorie allowance for the day in one go. His constant criticisms should have been the red flag to leave. Instead, unbeknown to him, anxiety about my weight began soaring again. I started exercising more and eating less. Looking back, I can't believe how vulnerable I was.

Then, one day, the same man announced that he had googled me and didn't want to be with me any longer. He worried about what I'd be like on my bad days. I was stunned. I'd always tried hard to ensure my grief never became someone else's bad day, and his comment felt like a physical punch.

That night, I googled myself for the first time. Despite my determination never to be defined by past events, seeing myself through others' eyes was devastating. I had simply wanted to be seen as myself – a woman and mother with dreams and goals, not someone marked by public trauma, tear-stained images from a mass funeral and a high-profile inquest for my family.

Afterwards, my eating disorder intensified as I tried to make myself as small as I felt. I hardly recognise myself when I think back about it. The reactions of others to the failed relationship only deepened my pain. People's casual comments – 'Well, you're a lot to take on, considering your family history, aren't you?' And 'Who wants to compete with a dead man?' – reinforced my feeling of being judged and blamed for the trauma in my life. I felt I was seen as damaged goods.

By St Stephen's night that year, I was overwrought, broken and badly needed help. I had to face it: I was getting worse and wouldn't survive the coming year if I didn't do something about it.

I had always avoided talking about my eating disorder in therapy. It was my guilty secret, and I wanted to keep it. The disorder was a method of control in my life in a world that often seemed out of control. But now the eating disorder was out of control too. I turned to Dr Paul Gaffney for help, and he called upon Dr Paul Gilligan in St Patrick's mental health services. By the new year, help was on the way. I feel fortunate and grateful, knowing not everyone can access such expertise and care at short notice.

The team at St Patrick's wanted to admit me, but I refused to go into the hospital. I had Gary to care for and a job to hold down. So, they agreed to admit me as an in-patient on a home-care package. It involved endless Zoom calls with the consultant psychologist, occupational therapists and social workers. The nurses on the wards rang me twice a day, sometimes three times, depending on how I felt. And there was constant assessment and conversation. But I worked with them, and they worked hard for me, and the therapy I received was transformative in so many ways.

They made me recognise my constant efforts to make others happy and conform to others' desires. I was a people-pleaser who had to learn how to address conflicts head-on and say, 'It's not okay for you to say things like that to me. It's not okay for you to treat me like that.'

During treatment, I learnt that assertiveness often comes at a cost, particularly for women. When a woman sets boundaries and refuses to accept disrespect she may be labelled difficult or damaged. When she chooses to move on from people who do not deserve her time or headspace, she's labelled contrary, damaged or plain crazy.

The team at St Patrick's helped me understand that my reactions to trauma were normal, explaining the psychological and physiological impact of the fight-or-flight response and validating my experiences. They gave me tools to recognise triggers and cope with overwhelming emotions.

While I acknowledge that my eating disorder and PTSD will always be part of my life, I've developed strategies to challenge triggers and assert myself in stressful situations instead of withdrawing and self-harming.

The eating disorder remains a constant presence. I study old photos of myself looking gaunt and wonder how I ever thought I was overweight, yet still feel that pull towards unhealthy behaviours. The internal conflict can be lonely, and the disorder resurfaced in 2024 after another traumatic personal period in my life.

Once again, I went back down that rabbit hole of not eating and over-exercising. It was another case of 'burn to learn'. I habitually learn through making mistakes but at least I always gain valuable knowledge from these setbacks.

This time, I found an extra source of support through fitness professionals, like Adrian McDonnell of McLifestyle Fitness. My coaches, Kevin and John, have also been transformative. Their non-judgemental approach and consistent encouragement have helped reshape my self-image and relationship with nutrition. Adrian wisely noted at the start of 2025, 'People above you will never try and bring you down' – a simple but powerful truth.

Cruel words are especially magnified when living in small communities. I still think back to that #Istandwith castlerahanns post on Facebook. And that vile comment about Richie that someone made in my past. I urge people to be cognisant of their words and behaviours towards others. No one should underestimate how their words, actions, and airing of personal opinions on social media can affect and injure others, especially those already wounded or traumatised.

Very dark things have happened, and I've worked hard to survive them. However, throwaway comments, casual abuse, attempts to isolate and irresponsible actions by other people, including a relentless smear campaign, pushed me close to the edge at times.

Thanks to the team's help at St Patrick's, I recognise judgement and harsh words for what they are – a reflection of the people who air these feelings rather than anything to do with me. I now have enough self-esteem and confidence to say, 'Well, that's your problem, not mine. If that's your mindset, it's your issue.'

I've learnt that I don't need other people to validate my feelings. And I don't need other people to tell me I'm good enough. Dr Paul Gaffney turned my life around by helping me process my traumatic past. Intensive treatment at St Patrick's hospital helped me with my eating disorder and gave me life skills for the future. Working with health and fitness professionals has also been uplifting and enlightening. Many people have helped me heal and given me the coping strategies to become stronger. Many women in my life have empowered me to progress in my career, especially in recent years. As a result, a lot has changed for the better.

I poured my heart into finishing my studies for a master's degree in human resources management. My thesis, 'The Possible Existence of Vicarious Trauma among Healthcare Employees in Ireland', focused on a subject I know a lot about. I used research to shine a light on the risk to employees who are constantly exposed to other people's trauma and the implications for healthcare organisations in Ireland.

I was awarded first-class honours from the National College of Ireland for my efforts. As I wore my black master's gown and mortarboard cap, it felt like a personal triumph. I'd succeeded against overwhelming odds.

My career has flourished. I applied for a new job, went through an intense interview process, and am now an employee-relations lead at an acute hospital. Meanwhile, I started writing this book about our battle for justice for Clodagh and the boys. Everything has turned around and changed for the better. For the first time since 2016, I feel I'm somewhat back to where I should be in my life and career progression.

Even though it's an understatement to say my first serious attempts to find love again didn't go well, I don't regret trying. I've experienced emotional abuse, immature and cruel behaviour along the way, but I realise all of this reflected on those men and had nothing to do with me.

For my own well-being, I now understand that it is okay to cut ties with anyone who drains my energies and brings darkness into my life.

I have faced many challenges, including a distressing experience of narcissistic abuse. The truth is that trauma can often beget trauma, and I have learned the hard way to protect myself in relationships. However, the bad experiences have also led me to a greater understanding of how people can end up in relationship situations they never imagined. I'm glad to say I'm finally in a more positive and aware mindset where I'm more assertive about the kind of relationships I want and deserve.

These days, if I gift someone my trust and they break it, I walk away. I have stopped seeking the potential in people. Instead, I pay more attention to their actions and behaviours and what they consistently show themselves to be.

A man's behaviour will quickly reveal what he's about, and from now on, I will always believe what I see. My boundaries have been disrespected in the past, but thanks to learning on the brutal 'burn and learn' programme – I don't justify or excuse this anymore. Nor will I try to please someone who doesn't know his own needs, let alone mine. When someone lifts the mask and shows me who they are for the first time, I believe them.

From now on, I'll also believe the anxious feelings, the self-doubt, the low moods, sleepless nights and gaslighting. I'll recognise the tears, the mind-boggling mind games, the triangulation, the sickness in the pit of my stomach, the lack of appetite and the loneliness. And if someone says one thing and does another, I'll see this as a red flag and move on. If they try to define me because of the tragedies that happened to me, I'll turn the other way. I know my worth now and don't look back.

Critically, I'll believe that I cannot fix something I didn't break, and understand that if someone mistreats me, it's because of their own demons and nothing to do with what I've done or who I am. In future, if I want to experience a rollercoaster, I'll go to Emerald Park. I will sprint away from anyone who tries to undermine my happiness and independence.

Instead, I choose to believe in joy and excitement, the anticipation of a text, a call, a date, a hug, smiles, affection and warmth. I choose to invest my time in people who deserve it and genuinely reciprocate that investment. That in itself is healing.

I have my wonderful child, a strong, loving mother, a fantastic family and a close and loyal circle of friends who support me. I have a fulfilling career, great colleagues, independence, self-worth and happiness. I value what I have and have zero tolerance for anything that threatens it. There is no place in my life for toxic relationships, but I had to 'burn' a lot before I learnt this self-worth.

The foundation of all relationships is self-love – without it, we risk accepting less than we deserve. I've accepted in my life people who were a lot less than I deserved. My desire to fit in and 'to appear normal' led me to tolerate behaviour that I would never accept now.

As far as future romances are concerned, if someone comes along, great. If they don't, that's fine too. I sometimes miss having a partner and that sense of companionship, but it has to be the right person at the right time. I'd rather enjoy the peace of single life than let loneliness push me into relationships that harm my mental well-being. I have many more goals that I want to accomplish, and if someone joins me on that journey, it will be their good fortune.

I once felt cowed by fear that people might judge me for what happened in the past. I thought I had to work extra hard to convince people I was 'normal', unaffected by the catastrophic events in my life. Now, others' opinions no longer concern me. I don't apologise for my life or events beyond my control. I've grown beyond what's happened to me despite others' attempts to keep me in that box. My past experiences may have shaped me but won't determine who I am.

Some who hear my story praise me. They'll say: 'You're amazing. How the hell are you still standing?' My immediate response is: 'What bloody choice do I have?' My next response is that I have a beautiful son who deserves the best of me. I want to be strong for him and ensure he has a safe and happy childhood. A happy mother makes for a happy child. I also acknowledge that I'm still standing because I talk constantly and am not afraid to seek help.

Repressing negative feelings and fears is exhausting and stressful. Expressing such thoughts helps process those feelings, and by sharing them, I realise I'm not alone. I don't just talk about the negatives. I'm aware that I have much laughter and love in my life, and I appreciate and share all the good fortune I have too. It is important to be present and have gratitude.

Time has also taught me that healing isn't linear, and some days are harder than others. I've sometimes felt so hopeless that life didn't seem worth living. My saving grace was that I talked about my problems and wasn't ashamed to ask for help. Being open and expressing ourselves is crucial when it comes to maintaining mental health. Thankfully, the days when there was a stigma associated with raising these issues are almost gone.

For years, I wondered how I lost my little brother and husband without realising they needed help. Time has brought a deeper understanding of life and the acceptance that I wasn't to blame. I couldn't have known what was happening with them because they didn't talk to me. They were never open about their struggles or traumas. Instead, they internalised their feelings and never sought help.

I have learnt that strength is not about the ability to carry our burdens alone – it's about having the courage to share them with others. My sister and three nephews might be here today if Alan Hawe had genuinely opened up, told the truth without shame and talked. Instead, he only told lies. He went to his GP and never told her he was seeing a counsellor. He lied to Clodagh about what was going on in his life and ticked a box by seeing a counsellor. He persuaded the counsellor he didn't have a problem with porn. He wasn't using communication as an opportunity to get better but as a method to control and manipulate others. He saw us all as puppets in his little show.

The road to healing and making sense of what happened was hindered when my family's quest for answers collided with walls of bureaucratic silence. The original garda investigation moved to close the file on Hawe with mechanical efficiency. The perpetrator was dead, so there was no ongoing threat to public safety and no trial. Evidence was legitimately destroyed, the rest was sealed, and they closed ranks around uncomfortable truths.

But Mam and I needed to know what signs were missed, what systems, if any, failed and what changes might be brought about that could prevent another family's destruction.

I never wanted to face the media and go public with our battle. Neither did Mam. Trauma constructs its own walls as a shelter from pain, and it can be easier to live in emotional numbness with suppressed memories than to speak about them. However, those sheltering walls often become a prison, isolating us from healing and connection.

In the end, we had to break through the walls we'd erected around us and learn to transform personal anguish into advocacy. We did it because we knew we owed it to Clodagh and her boys to pursue the truth and to protect other women and children at risk. It took enormous effort and an entire new garda investigation to break through the defences of the original investigation and expose the real truth.

Healing is a long and ongoing road for me. Opening up in therapy, being honest and raw and exposing my vulnerabilities has not been easy. But once I started, it became easier, and the sense of relief when I now share a problem is immense. The greatest lesson I've learnt in recent years is the value of transparency, honesty and conversation. Talking about issues and breaking the silence makes all the difference. I'll always urge anyone in pain to talk and keep talking. I believe that's why I'm still here and so many others are not.

The past and the pain of losing my loved ones will always be part of my story but, as Clodagh advised, it should never define who I am or where I'm going. I can't change the past or bring back my big sister and much-loved nephews, Liam, Niall and Ryan. Neither can I help my much-missed husband, Richie, and my little brother Tadhg. All I can do is ensure their legacy lives on through the lessons they've taught me: that silence and lies can be dangerous, that connection is vital, and that by speaking our truth, we might just save not only ourselves but others at risk.

Today, I stand as a survivor and someone still working at overcoming the shadows of my past. By choosing to speak openly about my experiences, I hope to be a voice that someone else needs to hear and a voice that helps someone else. I know now that by finding our voices, we free ourselves and create spaces where others can speak up and move from isolation to community and from surviving to truly living. Every time I share my story, I hope I honour those I've lost and show others who are struggling that there is always hope, always a reason to keep talking, and always a path forward into the light.

AFTERWORD

10 March 2025

On a bright chilly Monday morning, I steeled myself for a last glimpse at the house where we lost my sister and nephews.

I hadn't seen Clodagh's home since shortly after her and the boys' deaths in August 2016. For me, it was a horrific crime scene, filled with mass murder, and I avoided the place that had held so many bad memories for nearly nine years. But today was the day when the 'house of horrors', as the media referred to it, was finally going to be levelled.

Gerry was already waiting as I pulled up outside at 8.00. The demolition crew was assembling on the site with the bulldozer and other equipment.

I'm still unsure what happened when I got out of the car because I never intended to enter that house again. But the front door was open and a shaft of morning light seemed to light up the kitchen sink where Clodagh had once stood. I could see her there before me again. The memories started flowing and all the years condensed into a single moment.

I saw Ryan pedalling furiously around the driveway on his tricycle with a Mohawk of spikes on his helmet. I thought of Liam with his PlayStation inside and Niall's nose buried in a book.

I realised that I wanted to go in. I don't know where the urge came from, but I needed to go to the sitting room where Clodagh had taken her last breath and say a prayer for her.

I felt myself trembling at the prospect as I told Gerry what I wanted to do. Dread had made me build a dark picture in my head of what lay inside. I had imagined shadows, mould, creaking doors and other physical manifestations of what had happened there. Instead, sunlight streamed through the bare windows, painting bright rectangles across the empty space.

It was the emptiness that struck me first – the walls and floors were bare, stripped of furniture and all the personal items that held so many memories. Gerry had cleared out all the contents in July 2024. Only some built-in furniture, empty wardrobes and a few cupboards remained. The silence also struck me. It was eerily quiet, just mine and Gerry's footsteps echoing through the place.

I entered the sitting room and stood in the spot where Clodagh had died. I intended to have a moment of quiet contemplation, but the intense rage that erupted inside me took me by surprise. The enormity and savagery of Alan Hawe's actions hit me again. *You bastard*, I thought. I walked through the house, tears brimming. The house was warm where the sun penetrated, but I shivered nonetheless.

I went upstairs but couldn't muster the courage to go into the boys' rooms. I knew their final moments were stained in blood on the walls and I never wanted to see that again. I was only in the house for minutes, but so many emotions and so many memories – both beautiful and horrific – ran through me that it was hard to know how I felt. I walked through those rooms saying goodbye, not to the house but to memories of my sister and her much-loved boys. By the time I reached the front door again, exhaustion had replaced emotion. I felt worn out, scraped clean.

It's surreal to see a house being knocked down, especially one with so much tragic history and meaning. All the calamitous noise and dust were mixed with disbelief and flickering memories. It was bittersweet. I felt that Mam and I had checked off another item on our eternal list of grief work, but it also felt like another part of my sister and nephews was being erased.

I also felt angry that they were gone, taken from a home they had never wanted to leave. I felt their loss again and the promise of all they could have been with the destruction of their house. I thought about how Clodagh would have thrived if she'd had the chance to leave Alan Hawe. I thought about the terrible loss of Liam, Niall and Ryan's young lives.

I worked that day, sitting at my laptop in the house of Clodagh's good neighbour, Edie, as the bulldozers reduced the house to rubble. It was difficult to switch off from what was happening outside. The thunderous rumble of brick falling, glass crashing and the cracks of wood and metal splintering must have been heard for miles.

When I emerged to the collapsed and broken shell of the house that evening, I noticed daffodils blooming at the edge of Clodagh's garden – bulbs she had probably planted. Something told me my sister wanted me to pick them for our mother. I returned the next day armed with scissors and tin foil wrapping to bring them home to Mam.

The demolition was a slow process that continued for days as the crew bulldozed the house, cleared the site and levelled it off. In reality, demolishing that house had taken years. We first had to conclude the legalities of ownership with Alan Hawe's family. Then, the application to raze the house was lodged with the council planners. It took eight years and seven months in the end.

I had expected a sense of closure, some definitive ending to match the massive destruction I had witnessed. Instead, I felt only physical and emotional exhaustion, and the dull acknowledgement of another task completed. The house was gone, but there was no clean slate, no feeling of the past releasing its hold.

Mam and I had initially planned to create a small public park where Clodagh's house had stood. However, she is a pensioner, and I am a single parent and a widow. After paying tens of thousands for the demolition, we realised we couldn't sustain the costs of landscaping and maintenance indefinitely. Unfortunately, the county council is not willing to assist either. As it is, we will have ongoing public liability costs and must fence off the site for insurance purposes.

Instead of the park, Mam and I decided to create a memorial wildland and small nature reserve on the plot of Clodagh's house. It will require less costly maintenance and provide a thriving habitat for wildlife. A horticulturist has already come to the site to sow grass and wildflower seeds, and Mam and I will install a memorial plaque there. I believe my sister would love the idea of new life emerging from a place of evil, death and profound loss.

My hope is that the site of their home will soon be transformed into a peaceful sanctuary and forever remain a beautiful and living memorial to Clodagh and her boys.

APPENDIX

Understanding Coercive Control

by Anne Clarke,
CEO of Offaly Domestic
Violence Support Service

Many people think of domestic abuse as black eyes and bruising, but not all abuse is physical. Only six per cent of intimate partner abuse is physical, according to domestic-violence expert Professor Evan Stark. That means if we look only for evidence of physical assault, we miss the other 94 per cent of victims who are experiencing other forms of damaging abuse.

Coercive control is a relatively new umbrella term to describe all kinds of abusive acts that seek to erase victims' freedom and strip away their sense of self. The term was coined in 2007 by Professor Stark, who widened the definition of domestic abuse in his book *Coercive Control: The Entrapment of Women in Personal Life*.

Coercive control is a persistent and deliberate pattern of behaviour by an abuser, designed to achieve obedience and create fear. This can include emotional, psychological, financial, mental, sexual and social abuse. Women are predominantly affected by coercive control, and for the purposes of this book, we are focusing on women's experiences.

The common aim of abusers is to dominate and control their victims. Through myriad tactics, they instil fear until the victims' confidence and self-worth are entirely eroded. They isolate the women, deprive them of independence and micromanage every aspect of their lives until they no longer have autonomy over their thoughts, behaviours or reactions. In short, their minds are hijacked by the abuser.

When women are subjected to coercive control, their daily lives are determined by the mood and actions of the abusers. Even if they are not physically assaulted, many victims live under the threat of violence. Intimidation is the main tool in the arsenal of weapons used by abusers. Many women talk about 'the look' from their abusers. The women may be in company or in a crowded room, but only they will recognise 'the look'. Once they see it, the women know their abusers aren't happy with what they are doing or saying and can expect consequences later when they are alone. After one or two frightening incidents, the women begin to self-regulate their behaviour because they know if they don't comply with their abusers' expectations, this leads to more abuse. The process allows the perpetrators to abdicate all responsibility if challenged about the abusive behaviour. I don't force her to do anything. She does it herself.

Knowledge is power, so abusers are likely to monitor mobile calls and texts and demand to know their victims' social-media and email passwords. They may also install spyware on the computer to keep track of women's internet access and review their browsing history.

Abusers use intimidation to keep women in a constant state of alarm and uncertainty so they never know when the next incident of abuse may happen. Intimidation can happen in the subtlest of forms in the home. Abusers may suddenly reach for something near their victims. They may stand up too quickly or bang a door. The victims are constantly on edge, unsure if this is anger and if it's directed towards them or not. However, the perpetrators are usually purposeful in everything they do. These unsettling actions are rarely by chance.

Intimidation can include threats to harm the women, their children or family pets. Abusers know that vulnerable children or pets are a valuable currency to achieve the desired outcome of control. They know women will usually consider their children's welfare when making decisions.

The perpetrators may first engage in a couple of test runs

of abusive behaviour. For example, they may kick the dog or 'forget' to give a child vital medication, leaving women fearful for those they care for. Abusers may also threaten to take the children for good and not bring them home when expected. Women will then live with heightened anxieties that their abusers may harm or abduct those they love. The perpetrators can capitalise on these fears and use them repeatedly to control their victims.

Once the perpetrators have established fear and intimidation at home, they will move on to isolating their victims from any sources of support. Abusers want their victims to feel totally dependent on them. They achieve that by making the women's world smaller, isolating them from their support networks. This may begin with barbed remarks about friends and family. The abusers make it difficult for friendships to continue by name-calling a woman's close friends or hurling accusations about her family.

The abusers make it difficult for the victims' friends or families to visit by creating a hostile environment. They may refuse to speak to visitors or join in family events. The perpetrators will assert, Your family hates me or They don't respect me. Don't bring them into my house again, or else ... The 'or else' – not knowing what may happen – may be all that is needed for women to withdraw and isolate themselves from their support network. They stop visiting their friends' and families' homes and engaging in gatherings in the community.

Until the perpetrators succeed in breaking all of the victims' ties, they will always keep the women close. Abusers will make it impossible for friends or family to have any relationship or alone-time with their victims. If a woman decides to call over to her family home, he will accompany her. He will go along if she meets a friend or family member for a coffee. If it's a girls' night out, he will demand to go or sabotage it: she will have to answer repeated calls or texts during the time away. This control may be disguised as I'm just checking you got there okay or Ring me and let me know how you're getting on. He may call and say one of the children is not well and guilt her into returning home because all they want is their mother. She may be instructed to send text messages to inform him which friends are in the group or told she isn't allowed to speak with other men while she's out. She may be ordered to take a photo of where she is to prove her location. She will be bombarded with interactions, and these commands from the perpetrator eventually wear the victim down, so she stops going out altogether. The rules of the game, as set down by the perpetrator, keep changing, so meeting people outside the home becomes more and more difficult. The easiest option for the women is pulling away from everyone.

Multiple pregnancies very close together is another strategy by abusers to keep their victims under their control. Having numerous children makes working outside the home difficult, so the women become even more dependent on their abusers. It also makes socialising or even leaving the relationship more complicated.

Over time, the women lose their connections with close friends and family and will feel trapped and isolated with nowhere to turn. The abusers ensure their victims will have nowhere to seek support and no outside influences. There is no one on the outside to observe or comment on the toxic nature of the relationship.

Women are often belittled, humiliated and shamed in a coercive controlling relationship. They may be told they are too fat and be forced to lose weight; as a result, they are always on a diet. They may be told they are ugly and lucky that their abusers are willing to be in a relationship with them. The women are often left in the dark about household decisions and told they are too stupid to have any opinion or say in what happens.

The abusers often control everything about their sexual relationship and feel entitled to sex on demand. Victims do not feel free to say no and can be coerced into partaking in sexual acts with which they are uncomfortable. They will comply under duress because otherwise they face the consequences. The abuser may become moody and difficult for days or hurl accusations of affairs and exhibit extreme jealousy. She may fear he will take out his anger on the children.

At the same time, perpetrators can have multiple affairs and blame the victims for their behaviour. Alternatively, they may deny these affairs, telling the women they are going mad and accusing them of being the unreasonable and jealous partner in the relationship. As a result, victims may feel they are going crazy and at fault for everything.

Abusers may control all aspects of their victims' appearance. They may insist their victims wear makeup or forbid it. They may decide how the women style their hair or what they wear. Abusers may control the women's wardrobes by buying all their clothes. However, they may disguise this pattern of control by appearing thoughtful and saying, I thought this would look nice on you.

They may also make women insecure about their own choices. For example, if a woman wears jeans or tight-fitting clothing, the abuser may say, I don't like that on you. You look ridiculous. You look like a prostitute. To avoid confrontation, the woman may choose clothes that she knows are acceptable to the perpetrator. Continuous belittlement ensures the victim complies with the abuser so that she can prevent another incident of abuse.

Financial control is a common tactic of coercive control. Women may be prevented from having bank accounts or forced to hand over their salary to their abusers. Some women must produce receipts for anything they spend. Perpetrators often run up large debts in their victims' names, damaging the women's credit histories and ensuring they cannot get future credit. Sometimes victims are given meagre budgets and are expected to pay all household bills, and for food, clothes and children's expenses. At the same time, the perpetrators place no restrictions on their own spending. The abusers know that women will find it difficult to leave the relationship when they have no resources.

A perpetrator may also stalk the victim before, during and after the relationship ends. They will just 'show up' at the same places to intimidate and cause the victim to be afraid.

Even if the women do leave, the lack of economic stability for them and their children is often unsustainable, and they will ultimately return to abusive relationships.

Systematic dominance erodes the women's ability to think clearly or to reach out and seek help. Perpetrators are also often very clever at concealing their abuse. In many cases, abusers will often be well-liked and admired in the community, so many women will feel they will not be believed and struggle to disclose what they are experiencing. Victims may see their abusers being held in high esteem in the community and feel shame and responsibility for the abuse. As a result, the victims will feel handcuffed to the perpetrator. No matter where they turn, their abusers have all the resources and supports, and the victims are braced for the next accusation or attack.

It's important to emphasise victims do not always recognise when they are being abused. Low self-esteem is one of the many factors that may make it difficult for the victim to identify coercive control. In addition, some perpetrators disguise their abusive acts with declarations of love. I only do this because I love you and want to protect you. Often, it's difficult for women to perceive coercive control as, intermittently, their abusers carry out loving and caring acts. These occasional shows of affection help bind them to the perpetrators as the women see glimpses of the attentive and loving treatment they encountered in the early days of the relationship.

Coercive control is often difficult to identify, so domestic abuse is far more widespread than many believe. One in three will experience some form of coercive control in their lifetimes. Creating greater awareness of coercive behaviours is important so we can identify the signs. Abusers can inflict severe harm and damage on their victims without lifting a hand, and nobody should have to live with constant fear, cruelty and tyranny in their lives.

Red flags for identifying coercive behaviour
- Isolating you from friends and family
- Depriving you of basic needs, such as food and medicine
- Monitoring your time, where you go, how long you go for
- Monitoring you via online communication tools or spyware; accessing your email and social-media accounts
- Taking control over aspects of your everyday life, such as where you can go, who you can see, what you can wear and when you can sleep

- Depriving you of access to support services, such as medical services
- Repeatedly putting you down, such as saying you're worthless or stupid
- Humiliating, degrading or dehumanising you in front of others
- Controlling your finances, giving you no access to bank accounts or running up debts in your name
- Making threats or intimidating you or harming your children.

Coercive control became a criminal offence in Ireland on 1 January 2019. The maximum custodial sentence that can be imposed by the court is five years. The Domestic Violence Act 2018 says that a person commits an offence when he or she knowingly and persistently engages in behaviour that:

- is controlling or coercive;
- has a serious effect on a person; and
- a reasonable person would consider likely to have a serious effect on a person.

The Act relates to tactics used by an intimate partner – a spouse, non-spouse or civil partner – now or in the past. You do not have to be in a sexual relationship for a partner to be an intimate partner.

The legislation explains that the perpetrator's behaviour has 'a serious effect' if victims fear that violence will be used against them. Also, if the perpetrator causes serious alarm or distress that has a 'substantial, adverse impact on usual day-to-day activities'.

Acknowledgements

To Gary: You are my world and my purpose in life. Your dear dad would be so proud of the young man you're becoming, and anyone who gets to be part of your life is privileged. You have more emotional maturity than anyone I know. Clodagh and the boys loved you so much, and she would be so proud of the loving, kind and empathic boy you are. You make me laugh every single day with your quick wit and pranks. Thank you also for your patience and understanding while I was writing this book and working on my thesis. I look forward to spending more time with you, making more happy memories and taking many more trips together. Love you always!

To Mam: Thank you for supporting me in writing this book; I hope I have made you proud.

To Gerry: The hero in our lives! You never want acknowledgement or credit for all you do, but I don't know what we would have done without you. You and Carmel are like second parents, always looking after Gary and me, and making every challenging time bearable. You're always there, supporting and helping us, and you'll never know how important you are to our lives. I love you both.

To Melissa, Audrey and Eileen: Thank you too for helping us to make more happy family memories.

To the many wonderful friends who have stood by me through thick and thin: Sinead and Saul; all of the Dunboyne ladies; Teresa, Niall, Lisa and Sharon, Chantelle, Celina, Caroline, Cathy, Clare, Kim and Linda – all of you have supported me, and I will be forever grateful. You have made me laugh, especially during the darkest and loneliest times. I have found safe refuge in our friendships and a place where I can be myself. Thank you!

To Kathryn Rogers, my ghostwriter: Over the last four years, we have formed a special relationship, and you will forever be my friend. I can't thank you enough for your patience and calming me at some traumatic times. We have had some really special conversations over our time together and, without you, this book wouldn't be where it is today.

To my colleagues and fellow professionals in the HSE: Your constant support and encouragement have been invaluable. I feel lucky to be part of a team where I collaborate with so many brilliant professionals daily. You have never defined me based on what has happened in my personal life. I wish to add special thanks to Gillian Ledwidge Dunne, for your encouragement and for instilling confidence in me. Also,

I want to add my appreciation for Colm Kinch: You have shared your wealth of knowledge and have taught me so much over the past two years. You have coached me to step back and see my worth, so I owe a special debt of thanks to you.

To the warm and wonderful community of Virginia: You welcomed us with open arms, and I am happy to call Virginia my home. Thank you for always supporting us through our grief and our journey for nearly nine years now.

To Dr Paul Gaffney: Thank you for being the healer I needed on this journey. Everything could have ended for me in 2018, but for you. Your compassionate guidance and expertise in your field have been invaluable to me. You have made a significant difference in my life and I will never be able to thank you enough for your help and dedication.

Anne Clarke of Offaly Domestic Violence Support Services: Well, we have been on some journey together! I need to thank you as a friend and as a great source of support during my own experiences of abuse. Your understanding, empathy and continued work advocating for women who are victims of abuse are inspirational. There are no words except 'thank you'. So many victims have been helped and saved by you, especially through ODVSS.

To Laura and Padraig McEvoy of SuperValu: Thank you for all you have done, and you know what that is.

To Dr Paul Gilligan, St Patrick's Mental Health Services: Thank you for your support from the beginning of our battle and for your integrity and determination to speak the truth professionally and personally.

To Tamara Downey: Thank you for your continued support and friendship on our journey.

To Claire Byrne, a media professional who works with grace and dedication and a lady through and through. You treated us with respect and advocated for us when we needed it most. You have no idea how much that means to us. Thanks also to executive producer Jane Murphy.

To Gavin Duffy: How can I ever thank you properly for all your efforts in coaching and mentoring us so brilliantly? You helped us navigate a media world that was so overwhelming for us then. Trying to steer me, in particular, was a challenge at times, but we did it with tears and laughter!

To Edie: You were a great neighbour to Clodagh and remain a great friend to Mam, Gary and me. Thank you so much.

To Kevin McDonnell: One random day, I rang you looking for a man with a van. I wanted to move the beautiful, nearly new piano played by Clodagh's boys. I wanted to get it to St Oliver Post Primary School in Oldcastle, where Clodagh, Tadhg and I attended. Without hesitation, you selflessly volunteered to take it out of Clodagh's house and deliver it to a school where it is now being used for the benefit of many children. We know that it wasn't an easy thing to do and we will always be grateful to you.

To Liam Keane & Partners Solicitors: Special thanks to Liam and Anjana Hanratty. Anjana, you worked tirelessly and professionally to ensure we were treated fairly. You have always strived for justice. Thank you for your constant support and kindness.

To Declan and Teresa Finnegan: Thank you for all your kindness and professionalism during a horrific time for us.

A special mention to former Minister for Justice Charlie Flanagan: Only for you, we wouldn't have had the opportunity to have had a Serious Crime Review or make changes through the Familicide and Domestic Homicide Review. You were the first to afford us the opportunity to speak and be listened to. I will never forget your warmth and kindness at our first meeting.

To Safe Ireland and Tearmann: Thank you for allowing us to participate in your valuable campaign against domestic violence and carefully and effectively utilising the funds we raised.

Thank you to all the teachers and friends at Scoil Chaitríona Naofa (Oristown National School) in Kells, County Meath, for commemorating Clodagh's life with beauty and reverence. Your thoughtful and respectful remembrance of my sister means more than words can express. Clodagh was lucky to have so much love around her, particularly from her friend, Ciara.

To Liam's friends: Thank you for always making ways to remember him, whether it be a song or a tree planted in his memory. It has been a comfort to know Liam was remembered on days when he should have been present at Virginia College.

To Professor Colette Darcy (formerly Vice-Dean of Postgraduate Studies of NCI) and Professor Jimmy Hill (former Vice-President of Academic Affairs and Research of NCI): Thank you both for giving me the opportunity to study at the National College of Ireland. Colette, without your support and friendship during the completion of my PGDip and MA, I couldn't have achieved all I have to date. You held me up in 2013 and encouraged me to keep going. You both brought big smiles to my son and me on graduation day and thanks to you both, I can be proud of how far I have progressed academically.

Former Minister for Justice Simon Harris: Thank you for actioning the next steps from the recommendations outlined in the Study in Familicide and Domestic Homicide Reviews.

To the head of the Serious Crime Review Team, Detective Garda Des McTiernan, the National Interview Advisor at An Garda Síochána, Inspector Brian Quirke and Detective Garda Michelle Wallace: Thank you for your exhaustive work and professionalism while conducting the Serious Crime Review from 2019 to 2024. You treated us with respect at every turn and ensured that every avenue of enquiry was exhausted.

To Adrian and John in McLifestyle Fitness: Thank you for

always encouraging me to be my best. You have both helped me rediscover my self-worth and confidence. Because of this, I am enjoying life to the fullest again.

Thank you to Rev Fr John O'Brien, PP Oristown Kells, for your friendship and support. To Rev Fr Dermot Prior, PP Virginia, who was the first one to visit my home to see Mam and I when we lost Clodagh, Liam, Niall and Ryan. We will always be grateful for your warmth and support. To Rev Fr Kevin Donohoe, PP Ballyjamesduff, for always giving such respectful and dignified ceremonies during the anniversary masses for our family.

To my publisher Ciara Considine, publicity director Elaine Egan, Sharon Plunkett and all the team at Hachette Ireland: Many thanks for your guidance and sensitivity while writing my book.